M000039326

I dedicate this book to my family and inspirational ideas that continue to guide me:

Since it is the will of the Almighty that our bodies be kept healthy and strong, because it is impossible for us to have any knowledge of our Creator when ill, it is therefore our duty to shun anything which may waste our body, and strive to acquire habits that will help us to become healthy. Thus it is written "take good care of your souls".

[Deuteronomy 4:15]

"May my love of the art of medicine inspire me to seek at all times to expand my knowledge and to see within each of those in need only the human being".

Moses Maimonides

To the love of my life and my wife of 24 years, Tracy. She is my trusted partner in all the things I do, and this behemoth of a project was no different. Her insight, brutal honesty, experience, creativity, and investment in the project were crucial in getting this book published. I could not have done it without her.

My amazing kids, Adam, Josh, and Gaby were always instrumental in keeping my stress levels down, as they often joined me for lunch as their school schedules allowed. Lunch with my kids has always been the highlight of my day, breaking up a long and challenging schedule of seeing patients.

THE BEVERLY HILLS ANTI-AGING PRESCRIPTION

ANDRE BERGER, MD

All rights reserved. No part of this book shall be reproduced or transmitted in any form or by any means, electronic, mechanical, magnetic, photographic including photocopying, recording or by any information storage and retrieval system, without prior written permission of the publisher. No patent liability is assumed with respect to the use of the information contained herein. Although every precaution has been taken in the preparation of this book, the publisher and author assume no responsibility for errors or omissions. Neither is any liability assumed for damages resulting from the use of the information contained herein.

Copyright © 2013 by Andre Berger, MD

ISBN 978-0-7414-9717-8 Paperback
ISBN 978-0-7414-8481-9 Hardcover
ISBN 978-0-7414-8482-6 eBook

Printed in the United States of America

Published August 2013

INFINITY PUBLISHING
1094 New DeHaven Street, Suite 100
West Conshohocken, PA 19428-2713
Toll-free (877) BUY BOOK
Local Phone (610) 941-9999
Fax (610) 941-9959
Info@buybooksontheweb.com
www.buybooksontheweb.com

FOREWORD

Nobody wants to get older. How can we take responsibility for feeling great and being happy as we age? Dr. Berger has the answers and solutions. He encourages us to live in health, take care of our bodies through exercise and diet, and learn about the details of our chemistry so that we can make smart, informed decisions about the best ways to slow down the parts of aging we don't like.

One of the first pieces of advice I got from Dr. Berger was the first day we met. "Are you happy?" he asked. "Happy and busy," I replied. I will never forget the words of wisdom he shared, "You need a sanctuary," he said, "and you can't just buy a place and call it a sanctuary, you have to live and breathe what a sanctuary means to you. Create it in your home and in your life. Live happy." This is the philosophy I found so refreshing and helpful. Live in the peaceful experience of your life and you will be happy. And healthy. And look and feel younger! What's right for you isn't necessarily right for someone else. Of course we all want to live longer, feel younger and look beautiful while we're doing it. Well, now we have a guide. At least I've never met another Dr. Berger.

Dr. Berger's book illuminates his ideas and solutions and backs them up with medical science and research. It's a great place to begin a program of conscious health. The next step is having a chance to sit with him and experience his wisdom one on one. I go to Dr. Berger and I advise all my friends to do the same. Dr. Berger is a life changer. You'll understand when you take the trip to Rejuvalife and meet him for yourself. I promise you won't regret it.

Cheers and good health,
Anne Heche

CONTENTS

PART III: ON YOUR WAY, PHASE 2

APPENDICES: CHALLENGES TO YOUR PROGRAM

INTRODUCTION

A BIT ABOUT ANTI-AGING MEDICINE

First of all, I do not believe we can live forever. What I do believe is that we can dramatically delay or even reverse the symptoms of aging. By doing so, we spectacularly improve the time we spend in this world.

http://www.youtube.com/watch?v=8QUiBAee6Ko

The medical and pharmaceutical industries have conditioned us to believe that these symptoms - low energy, loss of cognitive abilities, diminished sex drive, physical weakness, frailty, depression, and irritability - are an inevitable part of aging, something we have to learn to live with, something we should manage with medications. In my practice I have learned, however, that by not giving in to these symptoms we can continue to live vibrantly until shortly before our lives end.

This is the essence of anti-aging: to defy the common belief that we must face an inevitable debilitating decline as we grow older - and that it is normal. It is not.

This is not just my belief: I have seen it happen over and over again with my patients. We can maintain a state of youthful vitality regardless of our chronological age.

This book will show you how.

WHAT IS AGING?

http://www.youtube.com/watch?v=69VOS0J8M5M

To understand anti-aging medicine, you must first understand that aging is a natural process which can be influenced by many factors. Some of these factors can be interpreted as disease. I don't see aging per se as a disease, but rather as a combination of deficiencies and illnesses that break our mind and body down, over time, until they are ultimately fatal.

Thirty percent of what causes us to age comes from our parents. There is very little we can do to influence the genes we inherit, but researchers are working on it. The remaining seventy percent of what affects us is environmental. That, we can control.

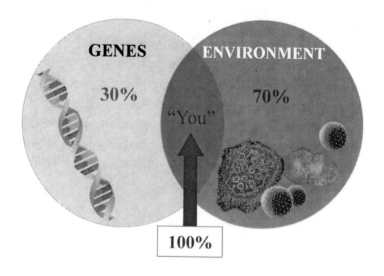

MANAGING OUR ENVIRONMENT

Exposure to sunlight, impure water, processed food, and toxic pollutants, along with the amount of sleep and exercise we get or don't get, all influence our genes. These environmental factors have a big impact on how our genes express themselves, for better or worse. Anti-aging is about what we actively do to make the best of the situation.

Think of your environment - light, water, food, air, and lifestyle - as a hearty, homemade soup. Many ingredients must come together successfully for the soup to be tasty and nutritious. Too much of one ingredient can throw the balance off. If you add too little of another, or add a wrong (or poor quality) ingredient, you would not want to eat it at all, and yet when all ingredients come together under the right conditions, the result is just perfect.

HOW TO MAKE CLEAN SOUP

A low calorie recipe for cleaning up your soup

INGREDIENTS:
• Commitment
• Proper Lifestyle

HOW TO:

Optimize lifestyle: exercise more, get enough quality sleep, reduce stress

Optimize Diet/Nutrition and Caloric Restriction: optimize nutrition and nutritional supplements, fasting and caloric restriction

• Reduce coronary risk factors	• Optimal nitric oxide levels
• Reduce inflammation	• Improve mitochondrial function
• Reduce oxidative stress	• Optimize hormone levels
• Increase oxidative defenses	• Exercise more
• Optimal blood pressure	• Get enough quality sleep

Our bodies are nothing short of miraculous. Every morning we wake from sleep, our feet touch the floor, and we start the day. It's only when something goes wrong that we begin to fully appreciate the complexities that occur, second by second, way below our consciousness; and yet it is awareness of our body's needs that allows us to improve its ability to function optimally.

For an anti-aging program to be successful, it is essential to improve the environment that our genes live in. If your soup is clean and robust, you have the best chance of aging slowly. When your soup is dirty, it's more conducive to negative gene expression and degenerative changes.

It's really that simple.

HOW WE 'TRICK' OUR GENES INTO YOUTHFULNESS

My approach at Rejuvalife Vitality Institute (RVI) is holistic. We treat the whole patient; medically, socially, mentally, and environmentally. It's important to understand my patients' genetic framework, as well as the environment their genes are in. Once we know this, we can go to work.

I begin with the medical basics. First I take a history of the patient based on a comprehensive questionnaire. Then I test the blood, saliva, and urine to gauge the 'markers of aging' and develop a status report on any obstacles to youthful aging. Together, each patient and I work to minimize those obstacles, and by doing so, avoid chronic diseases. We rejuvenate the patient in the process.

GENERAL PRINCIPLES ASSOCIATED WITH LONGEVITY

1. 80% Rule (stop eating when you're 80% full)
2. Plant Power (more veggies, less protein and processed foods)
3. Red Wine (consistency and moderation)
4. Plan de Vida (know your purpose in life)
5. Beliefs (spiritual or religious participation)
6. Down Shift (work less, slow down, rest, take vacation)
7. Move (find ways to move mindlessly, make moving unavoidable)
8. Belong (create a healthy social network)
9. Your Tribe (make family a priority)

Blue Zone Longevity Locations around the World:
- Costa Rica
- Japan
- Okinawa
- Sardinia
- Loma Linda, California

My practice at RVI treats patients of all ages, with most ranging from forty to eighty-five. Younger clients are usually suffering from a challenged ability to keep up in modern society. They have lost their energy. Simply put, they just don't feel right - this feeling is epidemic in today's world. Older patients' symptoms range from an inability to sleep and loss of sex drive, to loss of vitality and depression that often comes with aging; these symptoms are also epidemic.

There are various causes for a loss of vitality. For younger people it is frequently a matter of an unhealthy lifestyle; long work hours, little sleep, bad diet, alcohol and/or drug abuse. These drugs are often pharmaceuticals prescribed for one condition or another that have been used as a Band-Aid to mask an underlying, often very treatable, condition. For older adults it's usually a combination of these same issues, coupled with hormonal decline.

In addition, older people frequently develop depression that coincides with the loss of their youthful appearance. Most of my patients come in with a host of concerns such as wrinkles, sagging skin, skin pallor, disappearing body contours, and hair dullness or loss. These physical symptoms of aging tend to create a loss of self-esteem.

The good news is that we're now beginning to understand some of the complexities of the aging process. We are learning more from a biological perspective, especially about the need to maintain youthful hormone levels. Most importantly, we are learning even more about how much can be gained from behavior changes alone. I've learned so much from my patients, and wanted to share my findings. We'll explore both sides of the anti-aging coin: what we can do to mitigate or reverse the effects of aging in terms of behavior, and what we can do from a biochemical perspective.

HOW WE TURN BACK THE CLOCK

The way we live our lives contributes greatly to how we age. It's no surprise that the basis of all anti-aging medicine is changing behaviors and habits. Without proper attention to how we eat, sleep, exercise, and cope with stress, we will not have the proper foundation for the multitude of chemical and cosmetic changes that make up an effective anti-aging therapy.

http://www.youtube.com/watch?v=hUbPBp0Maqk

We understand certain concepts about health intuitively. Sometimes they are part of our social or evolutionary history. Although it isn't always the case, most of what scientists have discovered about the impact of behavior on health and aging coincides with our intuitive sense of what is good for us. It is important for doctors to validate what is true in each case. In the end, though, it turns out that simple behaviors - eating, exercising, sleeping, and dealing with stress - have important biological impact. These behaviors affect the rate at which we age.

There are four foundational components to the RVI anti-aging program. As the founder of Rejuvalife Vitality Institute I designed this program, and I often liken these four components to legs on a table. If one is missing or imbalanced, the table will lean or fall over. If all are strong and balanced, the table will hold up most anything. The four legs to my anti-aging foundation are: nutrition, exercise, sleep, and stress. All are important, and each needs to be addressed.

Nutrition

Your body must be adequately nourished to function optimally, so it should come as no surprise that the first leg to our table is a nutritionally balanced diet. Together we will evaluate and discover what nutrients your body is lacking, as well as what it may have in excess. We then create an eating plan to meet your individual needs.

For many patients, the first thing we address is quantity. Most adults simply eat too much. When you want to develop a more ideal body composition - changing fat to muscle and moving into a normal weight range usually starts with reducing calories.

We want calories that contribute to anabolism, the creation of healthy tissue, so I encourage healthy calories.

The first priority is to eat less. We must then eliminate bad stuff like saturated fat and worthless carbohydrates. Our next focus is on eating more good stuff, such as vegetables, and also making sure you consume an adequate amount of protein. There are other things to examine, including the balance between fat and protein, but overall it's about eating less and eating healthy in ways that are both intuitive and scientific. Organic whole foods, whole grains, and vegetables are key, and I'll explore this in more detail later on.

Exercise

Exercise is the next leg, and it's crucial. Biologically we are designed to move, and how we move, both the quality and quantity, is a critical aspect of aging. A sedentary life is a huge contributor to the aging process. Many people say they don't like to exercise, but often find that once their nutritional needs are met, they have more energy to work out and enjoy it much more. As we age, cardiovascular health, muscle mass, balance, and flexibility deteriorate. Most of us need the triad of regular cardiovascular conditioning, muscle training, and flexibility/balance routines.

Good nutrition and exercise go a long way toward maintaining and restoring youthful cardiovascular health, muscle mass, balance, and flexibility. Together, diet and exercise will maintain energy and slow down the aging process while creating a normal, healthy body composition.

Sleep and Stress Management

The last two legs of our table are sleep and stress management. To put it simply, you will never be successful with anti-aging, let alone be healthy, if you do not get enough restful sleep; and you will never slow down the ravaging effects of aging if you are trapped in a world of stress. These are the third and fourth legs on which we build the anti-aging foundation.

Once the foundation of nutrition, exercise, sleep, and stress management is firmly in place, we can focus on the biochemical aspects of aging and what can be done to slow down or reverse any symptoms.

Hormone Replacement

One of the central themes in anti-aging medicine is that as humans age, we experience a decline in most of our hormones. We also experience an increase in some, but they are mostly destructive. All together, the hormonal shift in our bodies is catabolic, meaning it contributes to a breakdown of tissue, rather than anabolic, which builds tissue.

You might ask, "which is the chicken and which is the egg? Are declining hormones the cause or the result of aging?" These are good questions, but from an anti-aging perspective, it doesn't really matter. In the end, what matters are the symptoms. Hormones are vital to the positive buildup and maintenance of human organs and tissue, and declining hormones play a big part in the breakdown and deterioration of the human body.

We treat this decline as a deficiency disease. Some of the signs and symptoms of aging, such as moodiness, lower sex drive and energy levels, and frailty, can be corrected with hormone replacement. In addition to mitigating the symptoms of aging, proper hormonal balance can help prevent chronic disease, but only if accomplished in conjunction with an optimal lifestyle.

All of the elements of a successful anti-aging program need to be implemented simultaneously. Good nutrition, followed by exercise, proper sleep, stress reduction, and the correction of hormone deficiencies will work together to create a healthy, happy, more youthful you.

A LITTLE EXTRA HELP: AESTHETIC CHANGES

Finally, there is the matter of appearance. Many patients come to my office at RVI because they look in the mirror one day and don't like what they see. Appearance is certainly one of the major signs of aging. While looking older is natural, we still want to look as young as we feel. The mindful combination of the aforementioned legs of anti-aging is what will have the greatest impact on achieving a youthful look.

Anti-aging medicine is our ability to change our present circumstances in terms of behavior and biochemistry, but we are also trying to compensate for a person's history of aging, especially if they are older. While anti-aging therapies can reverse many things, sometimes dramatically, there are signs and symptoms of aging, such as wrinkled skin and skin laxity (looseness), that call for cosmetic procedures.

In general, looking good is affected far more by how we live than by anything we can do with cosmetic procedures. The best cosmetic therapy is meant to improve the way we live and how we deal with toxins in our environment.

Changing Habits

Anti-aging is a lifelong process. The goal is to maintain an optimal lifestyle throughout your years. How much effort you must put forth depends on your individual needs. You may only require a modest lifestyle adjustment and an occasional check-in, or you may have

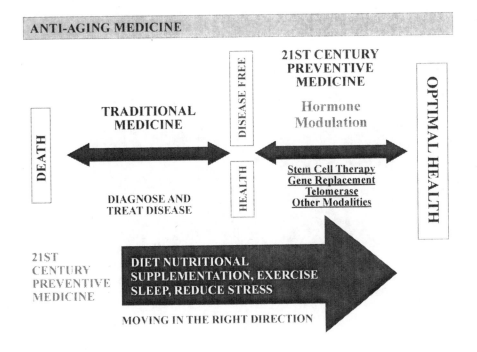

hormonal issues that require a more comprehensive treatment program. Either way, there is no universal end point.

This is not a negative prognosis. To say there is no end point to the practice of anti-aging is another way of declaring the fundamental aim of anti-aging medicine: to extend the experience of wellness into the final decades of our lives.

We all must be active participants in this lifelong journey, so that we can thrive well into our older years.

* * *

It is often said that a picture is worth a thousand words, so before I jump into discussing my RVI treatment protocol, I thought it might help to share the success stories of two of my patients, Marie Miano and Rob Richards. Both Marie and Rob came to me with many symptoms of premature aging. I worked together with each of them and we were able to reverse many of their symptoms, dramatically improving their health, vitality, and appearance. The following are their stories, as told by JP Faber, the former editor of New You Magazine..

Success #1: Marie Miano

MARIE BEFORE AND AFTER

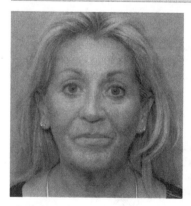 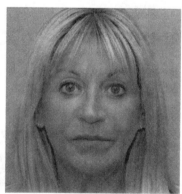

BEFORE   AFTER

Marie Miano is in her late fifties: a successful entrepreneur with homes in Southern California, upper New York State, and the Caribbean. She and her husband own nineteen IHOP restaurants in the United States.

Marie came to Dr. Berger in 2007. She was suffering from menopause, depression, low energy, mood swings, and no sex drive. She also had problems sleeping, and was overweight. I met Marie in her home in Santa Clara, California, four years after she had become Dr. Berger's patient. She came to the door in black shorts, high-heeled boots and a low-cut top. She looked to be somewhere in her forties and was bursting with energy.

This was a far cry from the obese, depressed person she describes herself as having become, the result of long hours and years of work as an accountant, combined with smoking, no exercise, and lots of bad food. "Normal for me was working anywhere from seventy to ninety hours a week, especially during tax season," she told me. "There were times that I would work at my desk until I fell asleep on my keyboard."

Marie had developed lots of bad habits that left her not only exhausted, but obese. "How do you maintain your energy to work if you're always tired? By eating junk food," she said. "You do what you have to do, so you develop very bad eating habits. You call up and get takeout food all the time. You eat the wrong things."

By the time Marie met Dr. Berger she had already lived in Los Angeles for fifteen years. This was after having moved from New York, where she'd been an accountant for Prudential and Borg Warner. Her husband had been transferred to Southern California as corporate operations director for IHOP. Marie started her own accounting firm in LA for small companies, then worked with her husband when they started to acquire IHOP franchises a few years later.

By the time Marie met Dr. Berger she had also had LAP-BAND® surgery, something she and her husband had decided to do the year before.

"It was New Year's and my husband and I were sitting on the couch. His father had died three years before, his mother had died, my father had died, and my mother had cancer. We looked at each other and said, 'if we don't do something now we'll be just like everyone else [in the family].'" After doing a lot of research to find the right surgeon, Marie and her husband flew to Mexico for the LAP-BAND® surgery, which was successful for both of them, but despite her weight loss (though she still had some to go) she wasn't feeling good.

"By then I was already going through menopause. Everything else in my life was supposed to be good. We were doing well in business, but health-wise I felt like garbage. I was sitting in [another doctor's] office one day and read Suzanne Somers book. That started it. I borowed the book from the doctor and kept it. I read every page and said, 'That's me!' And that's how I found Dr. Berger. His name was in the book."

The book that Marie read was one of a series written by Somers describing her transformation to a younger, more vibrant and sexy self via hormone replacement therapy and other anti-aging procedures.

Marie describes herself at that time as a woman who had become listless about life.

"With all the success we'd had in business, we agreed I could semi-retire at fifty-five, but I didn't want to do anything. I wasn't happy, I wasn't feeling good, and even though I had lost a lot of weight, I had no energy. I couldn't sleep. I had every symptom known to mankind," she says. She was also smoking as much as ever.

"Walking into Dr. Berger's office and sitting with him for the first time, I basically broke down and told him, 'I don't know what it is. I don't know what the problem is. I can't sleep. I don't have any energy...' And he said, 'I can help you.' I had also been a smoker for more than forty years, and Dr. Berger said the first thing I was going to do was quit smoking. I laughed at him." Marie took Dr. Berger's advice and went to a laser center that specializes in the use of laser beams (instead of acupuncture needles) to stimulate certain nerve centers that help block sensitivity to - and hence cravings for - nicotine. In Marie's case, it worked.

"I told Dr. Berger that I'd tried everything known to man, that it's not going to ever happen. He sent me to this place and in half an hour I'd quit smoking. I mean, I walked in and half an hour later I came out a non-smoker, and I haven't touched one since. It was the most amazing thing," said Marie. The laser acupuncture was followed by a course of supplements for detoxification, which she took for about a month afterwards. She said, "I never had one withdrawal symptom."

That was one of the first steps to Marie's individual anti-aging program from Dr. Berger and RVI, along with testing Marie for food sensitivities, hormone imbalances, and vitamin deficiencies. The next step was getting her to exercise. "I literally, at that time, could not walk for more than ten minutes, and that was even after losing weight. I couldn't breathe, didn't have the energy, nothing." Dr. Berger started her small, adding just a minute a day.

"He said, 'I'm not asking you to do a lot. All I want you to do is walk for fifteen minutes tomorrow, then the next day walk sixteen minutes.' And I did. I walked slowly. I had to be the slowest walker in the whole world, but I said, 'Okay, we're going to try this,' and after two months I was walking for an hour a day."

Marie said when we met that she now walks six miles a day, at a pace of about four and a half miles per hour. "I do a fast walk, plus some weights and things like that, and I could go forever. People call me the Energizer Bunny now. I have so much energy, it's incredible."

Next came Marie's re-education in terms of diet, and adopting Dr. Berger's recommendations for increased intake of vegetables and fruits.

"I'd been on the diet roller coaster for thirty years, and gave up when I crossed two hundred pounds," Marie admitted, which was heavy for her 4' 11" height. "That was in 2006. My husband was over three hundred pounds, and that's when we both decided to go to Mexico together and have the surgery."

Marie said she'd tried previous diets, but they'd never held. "Any diet that I had been on in the past, I was always successful, I always lost the weight, but it never made a difference because within three months I was right back where I'd started, plus had gained more weight. I went on Oprah Winfrey's Optifast® diet, I was on Medifast®, I was on Fen-Phen, I took diet pills, I did Slim-Fast®. You name it, any one that's been out there, whether in the mail or in the grocery store, I tried everything; and every one of them worked, but they don't keep working unless you change your life."

What made the difference this time was just that, a life with new habits. "This was a total changing of my life. Now, although I still do eat junk on occasion, I've changed a lot of my habits and make better choices for myself. I have committed myself to getting healthy. After getting into exercising I decided that if I want to eat, I'm going to eat, but I am going to work off every single calorie that I stick in my mouth, and since I don't want to work out all day long, I need to be conscious of what I'm putting in there. I pay attention to what I'm doing now, for myself and for my family, and I try to go back to more [natural things], and not eat so much packaged food."

Knowledge about herself has been another one of Marie's most powerful tools.

"Dr. Berger tests your body for allergies, which can include foods not necessarily bad for you, like spinach. Spinach was one of my favorites and an exceptional food, but not a good food for me," Marie said. "You find out which foods are making you feel bad, leaving you with no energy, making you feel tired, or generally making you not feel well. When you have your own personal list of what to avoid or eat less of, that is a huge help. Half the battle is knowing the source of your problem, what's causing it, and what to do about it. It also helped that all the testing was done right at the Rejuvalife Vitality Institute (RVI), Dr. Berger's practice in Beverly Hills. I didn't have to race around to multiple labs and appointments. Dr. Berger made the process easier than I could have imagined."

Marie also became a dedicated consumer of supplements and vitamins. Every two months she assembles all of the supplements prescribed by Dr. Berger, and puts them into daily packets of pills.

"It can be time consuming and it can be expensive, but I have to say, I'm a relentless pill taker now. My husband says I'm nuts, but the difference from four years ago to now is thirty years in the way I feel, and if that's all it takes, along with the other changes, then it's well worth it," Marie said.

Her only doubt, she confessed, was worries about hormone replacement therapy. "One month I would hear on the news how hormones were great, how hormone replacement therapy was wonderful. The next thing was that it causes cancer, or something else." What finally convinced her was the research on bio-identical hormones, distinct from the synthetic hormones used in studies that questioned the safety of hormone replacement therapy. "What these hormones do is try to bring your body back to its thirties, when it was most protected from these diseases [of aging]."

Marie said she now sees hormone replacement as dealing with fundamentals, rather than responding to symptoms. "I have some friends who go to the doctor because they get depressed, and they get an antidepressant, but they never address what the problem really is. To me it was far more important to address the source of the problem," she said. "Today I'm on a comprehensive plan and I've learned that you have to commit yourself to it, just like anything else."

One result, said Marie, is that she rarely gets sick anymore. "I think by doing what I do now my immune system is stronger and I don't have the same issues. Before, if anyone in my home were sick, I would get it. Or, if I had it first and they got it, I'd get it back again. The RVI program designed for me has made a huge difference in my body's resistance to illness. I haven't been sick in a year and a half."

As for the irony of owning so many IHOP restaurants, known for their pancakes and other high-calorie meals, Marie said, "I don't eat pancakes, and on menus you have to check the calories and fat. If you only eat the protein it's okay. It's just that anything in excess is bad for you. If you add a bottle of syrup on top of the pancake, you are adding another thousand calories to the five hundred you're already consuming. It's like McDonald's. If you are going to eat a Big Mac and fries and a 32-ounce soda every single day, you are going to gain weight. If you have it once a month, once a week, once in a while, it's a different ball game."

Today, Marie is a new person. She talks and gesticulates in an excited fashion: exuberant, and without hesitation. While she readily admits to a series of cosmetic procedures that brought her sagging body back to shape - a tummy tuck and skin-tightening common to people who undergo gastric bypass surgery - she said she is waiting for a stem cell procedure to restore a more youthful appearance to her face, rather than undergo a face lift. For now, how she feels is the most important result of Dr. Berger's anti-aging program.

"I'm fifty-eight, and I feel great. I feel like I'm in my thirties. I went from feeling like I was in my seventies to feeling literally decades younger."

As for the all-important issue of motivation, Marie said the entire anti-aging project was her own doing. It wasn't driven by friends, her spouse, or anyone else. She was tired of the way she felt, and unhappy when she saw herself in the mirror.

"I hated the way I looked, and I was sick of the endless cycle. You try to do something about it, you get frustrated and you feel like a failure... If you'd asked me twenty years ago if I would be doing any of these things now, I would have laughed in your face, but I've ended up doing it, and I've done it for myself. It isn't for anyone else, it's for me. When I get up and walk by the mirror and look at this person, I don't hate who I am anymore. This is the way I want to be, and I see this person every day. It makes me very happy."

SUCCESS #2: Rob Richards

ROB RICHARDS BEFORE AND AFTER

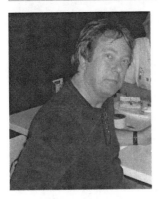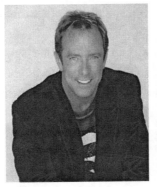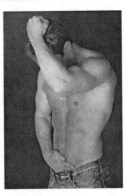

BEFORE   **AFTER**   **TORSO AFTER**

Rob Richards is one of only twelve people in the United States who can play the old-fashioned calliope organs that used to be in movie houses during the silent film era. For more than a decade he's been playing one for Disney in the historic El Capitan Theatre in Hollywood.

"Five years ago," says Rob, he suddenly felt old. "I was fat. I was sedentary. I hurt, and I looked terrible. I decided enough was enough.

I'd read about anti-aging and wellness, and the time was right. I wanted to reverse the clock."

Rob was fifty at the time. When I met him he was fifty-five, and hardly looked a day over thirty-five. His skin was rosy and young looking, his attitude joyful and optimistic, his body fit and chiseled. We met for lunch at Hollywood's famous Magic Castle, a Gothic Revival mansion that serves as an oversized clubhouse for magicians and those connected to the business. In Rob's case, his skills as an old-time organist gave him an entré vis-à-vis an old piano in the mansion that came with the legend of a ghost named Irma. He played the ghost piano from behind a curtain for a couple of hours now and then, but on this day he came to talk about anti-aging. Rob had discovered Dr. Berger after doing research online about medical doctors who practice anti-aging. "I specifically wanted someone on the cutting edge of anti-aging and wellness, including hormone therapy."

What Rob undertook was a complete 'lifestyle' program of diet, exercise and supplements, including rebalancing his hormone levels. The results, he says, "far exceeded everyone's expectations, including mine."

Today, in addition to being a musician, Rob is a male model. His portfolio of photos shows a cut and ripped man who looks decades younger than his actual age. "I have been completely transformed and become a different person. The biggest surprise is that in my fifties I have a better body than I did in college. I am able to train like a twenty year old athlete in the gym, I am better able to withstand stress, and my libido is like a teenager's."

When Rob came to see Dr. Berger, he had the problems common to men hitting the mid-century mark - low testosterone, irritability, and out-of-control stress that was taking a toll on his health and body. Among other things he was in the first phases of a tough divorce and a major lawsuit regarding the production of a television show.

Right from the start, Rob confessed that he was not perfect, and in fact deeply appreciated Dr. Berger's eighty/twenty concept - that you have to be able to slack off and have a little fun some of the time.

In Dr. Berger's words: "I first encountered this idea from a fellow named Bill Phillips in a program called *Body for Life*, but that was slightly more from a body building angle. Phillips' theory was that if you are strict with your diet six days a week, on the seventh day you can eat anything you want. It's actually good for the metabolism, because the body adjusts itself to a certain style of eating, so when you throw a monkey wrench in there, it goes, 'Wow, what was that?' and everything essentially resets." The same thing applies to body building itself, where you have to introduce 'muscle confusion' once in a while to benefit from your exercise routine.

Of course, slipping more than once in a while is deadly, and that is what had happened to Rob. "Like a lot of people in the entertainment industry here in L.A., I got so enmeshed in work that my healthy lifestyle and workout routine got away from me. At first it was not going [to the gym] on a regular basis, and then not at all, and then the diet started sliding because I was busy with work and travel."

Rob eventually found himself worn out by bad habits and a schedule that included playing the organ three days a week in L.A. and three days a week in Atlantic City, for months at a time.

Things came to a peak when Rob's back went out. After an intense massage at a spa in Atlantic City, he woke up to severe pain. "I think everything was so relaxed that the height of the pillow threw something out of alignment. Anyway I woke up in the morning with the most excruciating pain. A disc had slipped in my neck. I had never even imagined pain like this." Rob was realigned by a chiropractor who relieved the pain, "but it was a wakeup call to the fact that time was marching on and I wasn't twenty-four anymore. All this happened during the holidays, so it was a perfect time for a New Year's resolution - and I had heard about anti-aging and hormone replacement therapy, so I did some research and found Dr. Berger."

Rob says that Dr. Berger took one look at him and told him right away he'd be a good candidate for testosterone replacement. "And, of course, he was right."

Dr. Berger put Rob on a complete program of diet, exercise, supplements, and hormone replacement therapy. "It's truly multi-faceted, and really all about balance; not only hormones, but balance in life, stress, spirituality. It's about juggling all the elements of your life into an optimized lifestyle."

The results, which took about six months to fully manifest, astonished Rob. "I always like to say, it's not a miracle, but it's pretty darn close. It literally took fifteen to twenty years off of me, and it happened pretty fast. I'd say in about six months I saw ninety percent of what you see today."

As Rob sat and talked to me, I still couldn't get over the fact that he was fifty-five. He actually did look fifteen or twenty years younger, and I responded to him as such - as a younger man, much younger than myself, even though we are close in chronological age. It made me wonder, just what would it take?

In Rob's case, he attributes at least some of the success to his training as an organ player. "I'm very focused and disciplined because of my music work, so I went into this thing full guns. I don't imagine too many of [Dr. Berger's] patients take body building as seriously as I do."

The anti-aging regimen also led to a career change - or at least enhancement. "After getting the results that I did working with a personal trainer, he told me he wanted to put me in body building competitions. I thought about it briefly and decided it wasn't for me, but that modeling might be the thing because it has an artistic result and you work with great photographers and that sort of thing, so I went that avenue."

For his workout routine, Rob says that he maintains himself with four visits to the gym each week, doing about an hour of intensive training each time. He also walks every day for thirty or forty minutes, and takes a comprehensive lineup of vitamins and supplements. The key, he says, is to stay hydrated.

I always like to ask, if you could give one piece of advice to others, what would it be? "My advice is to drink as much water as you can," he says. "...and that takes discipline. I actually kind of hate drinking plain water, so I sometimes drink flavored waters, but you have to be careful, because they can be as sugary as sodas. I try not to do too many diet chemicals, because they aren't healthy for you; lemon is good."

Rob also attributes a lot of his sense of well-being to hormone replacement. "When your hormones are back on track, it gives you a general sense of well-being. You can't remember feeling that good until you get your body back in balance." To make sure all is well, Dr. Berger monitors Rob's blood on a regular basis; every two to three months. Using that as a guide, he varies the quantities of hormones like HCG and bio-identical testosterone so that levels are appropriate for Rob's needs and optimal health.

As for the supplements, Rob says, "It's a real jellybean jar full of things. I take a multivitamin, and I use Dr. Berger's in-house antioxidant. I also take Vitamin D, because there is a history of cancer in my family and I want to do everything I can to prevent that. I use what the health food store tells me is the finest fish oil there is, and I've been alternating it with krill oil, which is the latest and greatest thing." Rob attributes the successful lowering of his persistently high blood pressure to his regular consumption of fish oil and other healthy fats. "My last blood pressure test was the lowest it's been in my life."

Lower blood pressure is just one of the health benefits, distinct from appearance and energy levels, which Rob attributes to his anti-aging habits. Another is something often reported, which is an absence of routine illnesses like colds and flus.

"I absolutely never get sick. That's another miraculous thing about this. Literally, I only get a cold maybe every other year. It all works together in a systemic way to keep you healthy." Of course, nothing compares to the attention one gets from a revitalized appearance and looking markedly younger.

"I distinctly remember having a meeting with the fellows who run our Disney website. We were at lunch and this friend of mine leaned across the table and said, 'I don't know what you're doing, but I can't believe how you look. It's just amazing,'" says Rob.

What amazes Rob even more, perhaps, is how achievable his results are for the average person.

"The most remarkable thing about this is that if I could do this, then anybody can. The beauty of it is that once you get on the lean side of the curve, it's not that much work. The first six months are tough, and you have to say, 'Okay, I'm committed to this,' but once you get in the groove with it, even your palate changes. When you start eating clean and then you have the occasional greasy cheeseburger or plate covered with gravy, that heavy, fatty food just doesn't taste good anymore.

"The thing to keep in mind," continues Rob, "is that it's the combination of everything that makes anti-aging work. It's about balancing. If you take supplements but don't go to the gym, it's not going to have the same effect. There is a synergistic, bigger picture to it all."

As we left the Magic Castle, I thought how apropos that title was to what had happened to Rob. I looked at some of the other diners in the old mansion on our way out, and guessed that many of them were the same age as Rob, or even younger, and yet they looked haggard next to him. There was something oddly depressing and yet enlightening about it - all these aging magicians, ignorant of the real magic of self-transformation. If Rob could help it, they would all be patients of Dr. Berger.

"I'm so excited about what's happened to me that I'm like an evangelist. I want other people my age to know that we don't have to accept aging as a negative process. It can actually be an invigorating journey, as long as we have the right tools. That's how I describe my relationship with Dr. Berger. He's given me the tools; and yet, the tools by themselves won't do it. With discipline, focus, and work, plus the tools Dr. Berger provides at RVI, the synergy comes together for an exponentially rewarding growth experience.

"I think it all goes back to the sense of well-being. That's how I articulate it. I just feel better than I've felt since I was in college. It's about balance; whether it's hormones, exercise, spirituality, love or friendship, it comes down to juggling everything and coming out balanced, and the result is that I'm absolutely a happier person."

* * *

As these two success stories illustrate, Rob and Marie were able to reverse years of unhealthy living by following my RVI anti-aging program. These are just two of many patients who can attest to the almost-miraculous reversal of the signs and symptoms of aging, and many elements of the RVI program are featured here in *THE BEVERLY HILLS ANTI-AGING PRESCRIPTION.*

This book is an introduction to my RVI program, a guide to help new and potential patients better understand what they'll need to do if they make such a life-altering choice. Once you begin to understand the causes of aging symptoms, the balancing solution can and does fall into place.

Some readers will decide that I'm the doctor for them and will travel to my office so we can embark upon the journey together. Others will choose to take the information presented in these pages and work with their own doctor. While obviously I can only promise actual results to the patients I treat personally, there is a ton of information here that will help you begin your own path to looking and feeling younger than your actual years.

If you're reading this book, you've already decided to take that vital first step: educating yourself. Read on.

WHY WE AGE

CHAPTER 1

If we could stop the clock, wouldn't we? This subject has obsessed humans for as long as we've been smart enough to foresee our own demise.

There's no shortage of theories as to why we get old and die. According to the Old Testament biblical theory, we age and die as punishment for Adam and Eve's sin of eating from the tree of knowledge in the Garden of Eden. God's punishment was limiting us to a lifespan of one hundred and twenty years, though we rarely reach that age.

http://www.youtube.com/watch?v=KTM032v7Z90

In order to fully understand how we can slow the aging process, it's important to first understand what occurs as the human body ages. Contemporary paradigms of aging and dying come down to two basic concepts. There's the 'wear and tear' theory, as well as the idea that genetic programming is responsible for our mortality. The first school of thought says we get worn down from usage, like an old car, and one day stop working. The second school says that we are pre-programmed to age and die for the sake of the species.

According to the 'wear and tear' school, the culprits wearing us down include gravity. pollution, oxidation, inflammation, and radiation. These and other environmental factors all contribute to cellular mutation and collapse.

'WEAR AND TEAR' or GENETICS THEORY

A more precise, modern version of the 'wear and tear' theory pin-points the breakdown occurring in the tiny mitochondria within each cell - the microscopic factories that produce energy from oxygen and food. These wear out over time, which leads to apoptosis, or cellular death. So, if we could just prevent this damage from taking place, or at least slow it down, we would stay younger and live a lot longer.

From the genetic point of view, however, it doesn't really matter what we do. In the end, our genes control our fate. When we are young, our genetic programming makes our bodies grow to be strong, energetic and efficient. Then, when we reach a certain age, the genetic switch turns off and our bodies head south.

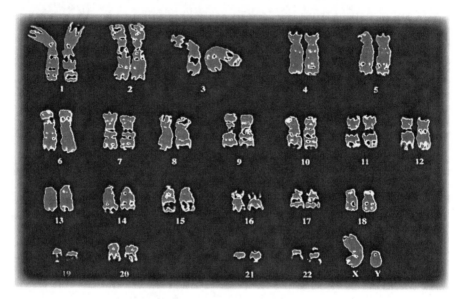

Chromosomes: Your Book of Life in 23 Chapters

The question is, if our genes control life and death, why would they 'choose' to kill us? Why not just keep us young and vibrant? The answer, says the school of genetics, is that we must age and die for the sake of humankind. It's all a matter of natural selection. In order to meet the challenges of a changing world, our species has to evolve, and that means passing on genetic variations to our children. Mother Nature chooses the best of the bunch. Once we've passed along our genes, however, Mother Nature doesn't need us anymore. Old humans are sacrificed for the sake of the new.

'Wear and Tear' versus Genetics: A Little of Both?

Both theories have value, and both should be dealt with in any anti-aging prescription.

In terms of 'wear and tear', the goal is to change our environment and change our behavior within it. These sorts of changes are the subject of the first half of this book and of the RVI anti-aging protocol: how we must control what we put into our bodies (nutrition), how we routinely use and rest our bodies (exercise, sleep), and how we must moderate our interaction with the world (stress, pollution).

On the genetic side, we need to understand a little bit about reproduction in order to understand the strategy for mitigating the effects of aging. The survival of any species is dependent upon its ability to reproduce. Therefore, all of our best energy quite naturally goes into making us peak physiologically at the time when we're ready to mate, which for humans would be some time before our twentieth birthday.

Because it takes human offspring about twenty years to fully mature, parents can't just die off after reproduction. Biologically, parents need to be around and well enough to feed, teach, and protect their children. After that, beyond forty years of age, humans are pretty well redundant, and that fits with what we see, that the toll of aging usually hits in our forties.

From the genetic or biological standpoint, humans begin to decline in their forties, descending steadily until we enter a final decade or so of utter frailty and often, senility. As we will examine in the second half of this book, by restoring some of the chemistry of youth, we can 'trick' genes into avoiding what is believed to be the inevitable decline of health, and thus ward off many effects of old age.

Making the Best of Our Years

This is a fundamental concept for anti-aging therapies in general, and for my anti-aging prescription, as well. As human beings we have a limit to our lifespan. That limit is determined by the number of times our cells can divide. This is the ultimate barrier for longevity, because once our cells stop dividing, we die. For humans, according to Dr. Leonard Hayflick, this is approximately fifty times. Hayflick's theory, called the Hayflick limit, applies to every species, and it represents the approximate number of years we have on this planet.

For human beings, this biologically determined, maximum possible lifespan is about one hundred and twenty years, and if you look at the oldest humans recorded, that's been about it. If we had the possibility of living longer, there would have been older people recorded in history, even if only a few; but there haven't been any.

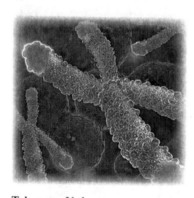

Telomere Nub

Interestingly, there is a physical marker for this age limit. It is called a telomere, and they are attached to every cell in our bodies. All of our chromosomes have telomeres, and their function is to secure the structural integrity of the chromosome. It's like an aglet, that solid little cap that prevents a shoelace from getting frayed, stringy, and useless.

The same idea applies to the human chromosome. When a telomere cap becomes thin and shrinks to a less than optimal size, it will affect the structural integrity of that chromosome, causing it to unravel in ways that will cause mutations. This eventually leads to an inability of the cell to divide or replicate, and this is cell death, or apoptosis. Ultimately, what it comes down to is preventing cellular death.

If there is going to be a major breakthrough that could increase longevity beyond one hundred and twenty years, it will theoretically involve some way to secure those telomere caps for a longer period of time. This is a major work in progress, and we're not anywhere near a conclusion yet. In the meantime, we are aging.

Anti-aging is not about living forever. It is about how well we age, which means maintaining optimal health throughout our lifespan.

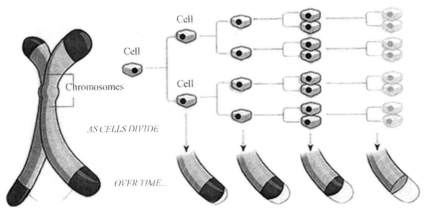

Telomeres, end caps that protect the chromosome

..TELOMERES SHORTEN, AND EVENTUALLY CELL DIVISION STOPS.

ANTI-AGING VERSUS IMMORTALITY

Anti-aging is less about pushing the theoretical limit of how many years we can live, and more about keeping us youthful within those limits. It's not about extending lifespan so much as extending our wellness span. You can also call it our feel-good span, as in avoidance -of-chronic-disease span, vitality span, or health span. Whatever you call it, the idea is to live at an optimal level of wellness, health, and vitality for the length of our potentially century-plus lifespan.

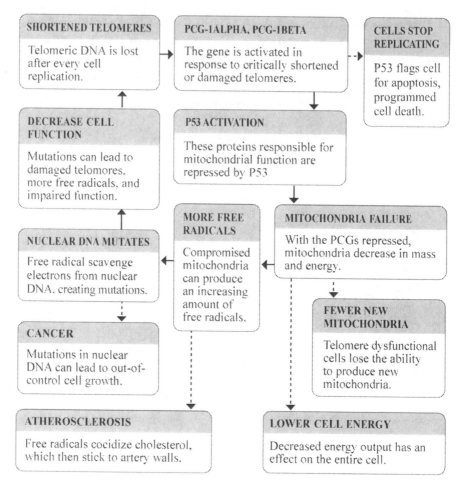

SHORTENED TELOMERES

Telomeric DNA is lost after every cell replication.

PCG-1ALPHA, PCG-1BETA

The gene is activated in response to critically shortened or damaged telomeres.

CELLS STOP REPLICATING

P53 flags cell for apoptosis, programmed cell death.

DECREASE CELL FUNCTION

Mutations can lead to damaged telomeres. more free radicals, and impaired function.

P53 ACTIVATION

These proteins responsible for mitochondrial function are repressed by P53

NUCLEAR DNA MUTATES

Free radical scavenge electrons from nuclear DNA. creating mutations.

MORE FREE RADICALS

Compromised mitochondria can produce an increasing amount of free radicals.

MITOCHONDRIA FAILURE

With the PCGs repressed, mitochondria decrease in mass and energy.

FEWER NEW MITOCHONDRIA

Telomere dysfunctional cells lose the ability to produce new mitochondria.

CANCER

Mutations in nuclear DNA can lead to out-of-control cell growth.

ATHEROSCLEROSIS

Free radicals cocidize cholesterol, which then stick to artery walls.

LOWER CELL ENERGY

Decreased energy output has an effect on the entire cell.

Uniform Theory of Aging

Aging as we know it tends to diminish the quality of life. Anti-aging endeavors to help us fight back and optimize our quality of life. Our goal is to increase wellness and vitality so that as we age toward our programmed ends, we can enjoy the best life possible.

I believe - and have seen in my practice - that people can remain vital right up to or very close to our final decline. The way this can be done is by cleaning up the "soup" discussed earlier - environment, nutritional input, and behavior - to every extent possible.

People must also understand their genetic predispositions as much as possible, then do whatever they can through lifestyle, diet, nutrition, exercise, sleep, and hormonal therapies, to up-regulate their positive genes and down-regulate genes that are, or are going to be, negative. That's the way they are going to have the best possible quality of life throughout their lifespan.

When it comes to living forever, the only immortal parts of us are the cells we pass from generation to generation. Only single cell organisms divide into new cells and continue to do so infinitely

The development of the human brain, a profound occurrence in and of itself, is a game changer in terms of anti-aging. Once you add thinking, creativity, and cognitive input to the mix, it changes the whole concept of aging. If human aging is just a biological phenomenon, then we need to take the thought process out of it, but as it happens, that is impossible.

THE BRAIN GAIN

Humans are certainly different from the primitive animals we evolved from, as well as other species that may be related to us. The brain rules us. What applies to other species in aging may not apply to us, despite similarities.

The fact that we live beyond our reproductive years, and even beyond our years of usefulness as guardians for our children, shows that our ability to grow 'old' relates to brainpower. Here, selectivity is based on the idea that a grandparent can help the family with his or her accumulated wisdom.

The fact that we can actually consider these theories of aging puts the whole idea of aging in a different light. Unlike other species, our brain tells us that we really don't want to be put out to pasture; we are going to do everything possible to prevent it. If we didn't have such a highly developed brain, we wouldn't even care. We'd be satisfied with our biological lot and wouldn't worry about taking care of ourselves.

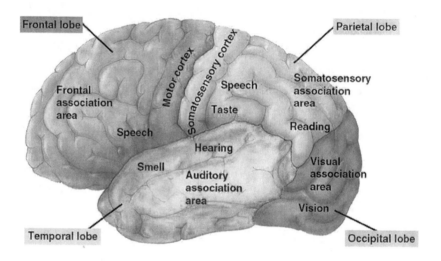

Of greatest importance is the fact that our brains and bodies are fundamentally connected when it comes to health and aging. This relationship between the brain and aging is not completely understood, but it plays a key part in the aging process. Understanding the brain's role is an exciting frontier in terms of understanding aging.

Let's look at the existence of human will, for example. There are innumerable clinical examples of patients surviving on the operating table because they refuse to give up, while others seem to have lost the will to live.

Why does this happen?

The human higher brain is a very important modulator of survival. The way we think, what we think about, and how we think about it, affects our health and how we feel. Depression and anxiety are examples of how psychological states can have trickle down effects with very real health consequences. They lead to biochemical and physiological changes that affect how we age.

Psychological states can either cause or reflect changes in neurotransmitters, creating changes in hormonal balances. Hormones then affect things like sleep, muscle mass, weight, and development of chronic diseases. It is all mixed in together - starting with what's happening upstairs - because the brain is so influential.

In practical terms, we don't respect our brain and its influence on health and aging enough. This goes beyond merely how we think, to the core of how we care for our brain. Proper health maintenance, to include whole body care, is as much about maintaining the vitality of our brain - the driver of our very being - as it is about caring for our internal systems and our appearance. These are things we must look at in terms of modulating the effects of the brain and controlling imbalances.

The good news is that this awareness of how the mind plays a key role in health and aging is part of treatment, with focus on holistic health and integrating the whole person - mind, body, and spirit. We now have a rudimentary understanding of what is energy based, as well as a primitive, basic view of what 'spirit' means in terms of brain function.

Eventually we are going to understand more about the energy patterns within us, which will be important therapeutically. Concepts such as energy meridians and energy-related treatments like acupuncture are gaining momentum in Western medicine. These types of therapies, along with practices such as meditation, yoga, and tai chi, modulate and balance the energy within us to make us feel better. When combined, they have an effect on the mind and the body as a whole.

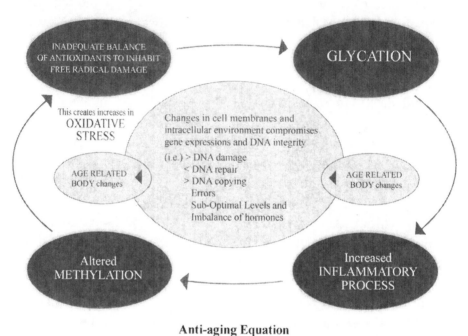

Anti-aging Equation
Each process sets in place a series of events that increases the other related reactions utimately causing a change in gene expression.

In the end, what we do with our minds extrapolates into body chemistry, physiology, hormone balance, and wellness. It is all connected. This leads us, and my practice of anti-aging medicine, to the idea that we must employ a holistic approach to each person. We are all complicated and there are many elements involved, all intricately inter-connected. A holistic approach addresses all relevant elements for each patient.

Something I found very discouraging as a young doctor practicing traditional Western medicine was how we often treat disease as a compartmentalized entity. Everything is a sub-specialty. As doctors we had to specialize in one field, such as rheumatology, cardiology, neurology, or endocrinology, etc. But humans are not compartmentalized; all of our functions are integrated, so while you may be able to treat a disease compartmentally, you're never doing the best job you can to keep a person well and actually prevent disease until you are stepping beyond compartments to treat the whole patient.

Health and aging cannot be compartmentalized, and neither can anti-aging. Our approach must be integrative. It must respect that we are all highly complex and all anti-aging therapies must work together.

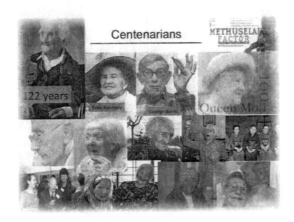

The best (and in my experience, the only) course is to approach both aging and anti-aging with a unified theory. That is the essence of functional anti-aging medicine, to look at how we function as a whole being. You cannot pigeonhole it any more than you can compartmentalize the human experience. It encompasses everything we do, everything we experience, and how it all inter-relates. That is the way I view aging as an anti-aging doctor, and this is what the rest of this book will explain in practical terms.

THE DOCTOR-PATIENT
RELATIONSHIP

CHAPTER 2

When a new patient walks into my office, I don't see a liver or a heart or a skeleton walking in. I see a very complex creature with a big brain that's going to take a lot of figuring out. I also recognize that this person is about to become a long-term partner with me in their health care and quest for youthful wellness. It's very different from how I used to perceive patients when I practiced medicine in a more traditional, compartmentalized way.

The first thing I do when I meet a patient now is gain an understanding of why they are here in the first place, and ascertain whether they are going to be a good fit for anti-aging treatments. We have an open discussion about their lifestyle and habits.

OUR FIRST MEETING

The purpose of the initial consultation is to think things through with the patient and decide if we are going to work together. This is a very important step, because we are going to get very close. I ask questions that are deep and personal. I will get to know them better than perhaps anybody else in the world. It's important for the patient to see that I not only share my expertise, but can also be a great advocate for them. It's important for me as well, because I stick with my patients for the long haul; I don't just see them for five minutes and say goodbye.

The reason I founded Rejuvalife vitality institute (RVI) is because it was never my style to provide quick, superficial healthcare. My professional mission is to really know my patients, because only when they feel totally comfortable with me will they let me in to truly help. At RVI I treat patients my way, and the overwhelming results we achieve speak for themselves.

Part of each first meeting is also to make sure that the patient's expectations will be reasonably met by this program, while introducing them to the program itself, how it works, and their role in it. I don't want anyone to get started until they understand what they are getting into, how they must commit to partnering with me in this, and how they must willingly comply with my guidance if they want their expectations to be met.

THE HOLISTIC HEALTH AND WELLNESS QUESTIONNAIRE

(SAMPLES)

Please answer the questions in each section below and total your score. Each response will be a number from 0 - 5. Please refer to the frequency described within the parenthesis (e.g. "2 - 3 x/wk") when answering questions about an activity e.g. "Do you maintain a healthy diet"? However, when the question refers to an attitude or an emotion (most of the Mind and Spirit questions, e.g., "Do you have a sense of humor?" the response is more subjective, less exact, and you can refer only to the items describing the frequency, such as often or daily, but not to the numbered frequencies in parenthesis. Be sure to add up your score for each section as well as you total score.

BODY: PHYSICAL AND ENVIRONMENTAL HEALTH

1. Do you maintain a healthy diet (low fat, low, fresh fruits, grains and vegetable)?
2. Is your water intake adequate? (at least ½ oz./lb of body; 160 lbs.=80 oz.)?
3. Are you within 20 percent of your of your ideal body weight?
4. Do you feel physically attractive?
5. Do you fall asleep easily and sleep soundly?
6. Do you awaken in the morning feeling well rested?
7. Do you have more than enough energy to meet your daily responsibilities?
8. Are you five senses acute?

TOTAL BODY SCORE _____

MIND: MENTAL AND EMOTIONAL HEALTH

1. Do you have specific goals in your personal and professional life?
2. Do you have the ability to concentrate for extended periods of time?
3. Do you use visualization or mental imagery to help you attain your goals or enhance your performance?
4. Do you believe it is possible to change?
5. Can you meet your financial needs and desires?
6. Is your outlook basically optimistic?
7. Do you give yourself more supportive messages than critical messages?
8. Does your job utilize all of your greatest talents?

TOTAL MIND/EMOTIONS SCORE _____

SPIRIT: SPIRITUAL AND SOCIAL HEALTH

1. Do you actively commit time to your spiritual life?
2. Do you take time for prayer, meditation, or reflection?
3. Do you listen to your intuition?
4. Are creative activities a part of your work or leisure time?
5. Do you take risks or exceed previous limits?
6. Do you have faith in a God, spirit guides, or angels?
7. Are you free form anger toward God?
8. Are you grateful for the blessings in your life?

TOTAL SPIRIT SCORE _____

TOTAL BODY, MIND, SPIRIT SCORE _____

HEALTH SCALE

- 325-375 Optimal Health
- 275-324 Excellent Health
- 225-274 Good Health
- 175-224 Fair Health
- 125-174 Below Average Health
- 75-124 Extremely Poor Health = Surviving

I always make sure to tell patients that there is really only one thing you need to do to be successful. You just have to do what I tell you. It's that simple. The people who do what I tell them will do well, and the people who don't, won't. They laugh when I say this, but in the end it's the truth. I can only advise a patient so much, and if he or she leaves the office and doesn't follow the protocol, they are not going to get the desired results.

In the first meeting I also explain a very important concept, which is that humans are dynamic creatures, not static, and therefore have ever-changing physiological demands. We're also individuals. Each of us is subjected to different things, such as different environments and stresses. These factors are also dynamic. So even when someone has made the commitment and begins the program, it's not necessarily going to be the same throughout the duration. Things change, and all the while, natural aging processes continue. This is why we need to form a relationship that will support and guide you throughout your journey, which is different from any other. I can't (and won't) just put someone on a program, then say goodbye and good luck, because it's only a matter of time before some fine-tuning is needed. Various changes are natural and normal, and we must be aware of them so we can manage them together, for success.

We begin working together by taking a complete medical history and doing some testing to establish what the patient's biochemical baselines are. I try to do a comprehensive workup, but also try not to overwhelm anyone. There is a balance between our need to get all the answers and the danger of burdening people with too much information at once. By its nature, the RVI program is front-loaded and heavy in the beginning. My patients need to learn a lot quickly, and then we spend a lot of time cleaning up their internal and external environments while tailoring a program to their own unique needs. Once we're underway we don't have to be as intense about it; we just have to make sure that the patient is maintaining.

WHERE YOU ARE COMING FROM

Before we do any lab tests, we gather a complete anti-aging social history. We want a lot of detail in this history because it reveals a tremendous amount about a patient's behavior, habits, and how they're truly feeling. This relates to and influences every area of anti-aging.

A patient's eating habits are only one example. Anti-aging is directly related to eating, and yet eating is often a social behavior, so if we put someone on a nutritional program, a.k.a. a diet, we want to know his or her social history of eating. What happens to them when they go out with a friend, or to a party? We examine how social environments change their level of control. We need to understand how they act in different situations, to see if they eat too much under stress, or too little, and so forth.

Taking a social history is fairly typical. Even patients of traditional medicine provide a medical history and go through a systematic review. It's just that ours has a different spin to it. I practice a form of medicine called functional medicine, which treats the whole body as one complete and integrated system, instead of a collection of separate parts. A detailed medical history at RVI covers all the critical health categories with a particular focus on function. We go through all the symptoms and signs of different organ systems in the body, with particular attention paid to the experiences we collectively call quality of life. This part of the review is time-intensive, and yet it helps me to best understand the patient and any health issues, past or current.

For women, we also take obstetric and menstrual histories while looking at female-specific medical conditions or events, and any hormonal issues. We examine things like the history of estrogen dominance, which is crucial to understand. For men, we look for things that specifically affect them - testosterone deficiency, for example.

Regardless of gender, we spend a lot of time on gastrointestinal history. The gut is a very important system. If you don't have a healthy gut, you're probably not going to feel well. It is essential in protecting you from underlying inflammation. If you have a gut that is not protecting you from antigens, foreign proteins, infectious agents, and/or toxic substances, or if you have a gut that is not assimilating nutrients effectively, it is unlikely that you can feel your best or function at optimal performance levels.

We simultaneously look at the immune system. It turns out that most of the immune tissue in the body - lymphatic tissue and lymph nodes - is located immediately around (you guessed it) the gut. In a sense, the gut is an immune-defense structure that protects us from the ravages of the environment, especially what we're ingesting.

As you might imagine, I always take a complete diet inventory. I ask patients to eat their typical foods for three days, then give me every detail about what they ate, how they felt after they ate it, what their bowel movements were like, and anything else they want to comment about.

BEYOND THE STOMACH

While the gastrointestinal history and examination of a patient's diet can reveal quite a bit, the human body is complex and many other organs and parts factor into our overall health.

The Mouth

Dental health is extremely important, yet often overlooked. It's clear now that a lot of dental issues, many of which can go unrecognized without professional examination, can lead to other organ system problems. We look for things like heavy metals leeching from dental amalgams. We look for

http://www.youtube.com/watch?v=1121U408TI4

chronic gum disease because this is a source of infection, causing chronic inflammation and sometimes a precursor to systemic organ failure.

Dental health is also essential for the proper assimilation of food. You must be able to chew properly because it's the first run at digestion. Chewing prepares food to the right consistency while the mouth produces key enzymes. People with poor dental hygiene may have lost teeth, an improper bite, or inadequate grinding motion. Each of these is a barrier to properly assimilating food.

Medications and Supplements

Naturally, we want an inventory of all medications, as well as supplements, vitamins, minerals, herbs, homeopathics, hormones, etc., that a patient is taking. We need to know this, along with any medical symptoms and toxicities they might have.

Family Medical History

In addition to the patient's own profile, we also want his or her genetic history - which really means their family medical history - to discover what could be passed along or make them more susceptible to disease. Family health issues often contribute a certain degree of stress, and some, if not dealt with, can become chronic and pervasive.

Lifestyle

Finally we examine the vast area over which we have the most control, and which is so influential - the collection of habits we call lifestyle. This has a powerful impact on potential for optimal wellness, because it dramatically affects quality of life. A great deal of the practice of anti-aging is devoted to improving quality of life. Indeed, this is the essence of anti-aging medicine; the idea that we can extend the vital, energetic, fully functional part of life. And yet, how many traditional practitioners of medicine make you fill out a quality of life/lifestyle survey? It's unheard of in most doctors' offices, but at RVI it's extremely important in our practice. Unlike traditional medicine, we

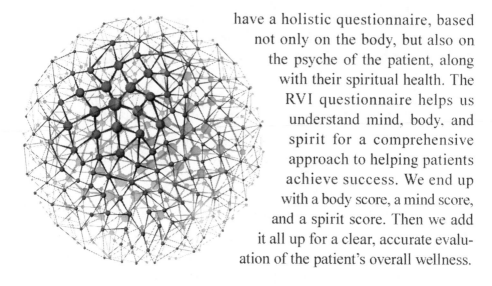

have a holistic questionnaire, based not only on the body, but also on the psyche of the patient, along with their spiritual health. The RVI questionnaire helps us understand mind, body, and spirit for a comprehensive approach to helping patients achieve success. We end up with a body score, a mind score, and a spirit score. Then we add it all up for a clear, accurate evaluation of the patient's overall wellness.

A MOTIVATED PARTNERSHIP

Finally, we produce a readiness assessment. This is just what it sounds like. It examines how ready the patient is to get started. I need to know the truth, so patients must be honest about this the same as when answering all the other questions. I ask for a number from one to ten on key items, so there is some flexibility - but it must be an authentic answer, not one simply put down to make me believe a patient is ready.

If a readiness score is low, I don't just turn any person away. I ask them to re-examine expectations, ability, and commitment, and we discuss again how results are based on effort. When a patient is fully committed, ready to take this on and be successful, they'll do what I ask. When they're not ready, they won't. I put that on the table. I'm not here to suck in patients and pretend they're going to see some magical cure. This is a process that requires both of us, working together. Anti-aging medicine is not like any other type of medicine in the sense that the patient really becomes a partner.

In the end, the treatment itself must be done by the patient. The foundation of anti-aging medicine is lifestyle. I can be the guide who provides the road map and answers questions, but if the patient doesn't do the right thing, he or she will undermine their treatment. Wellness doesn't come in a pill, or an injection. It comes from taking a comprehensive look at what needs to be done, and then doing it.

I want to know right away what motivates my patients. Some people come to see me feeling great, and just want to stay that way. Many celebrities want to remain on top of their game, with the goal of getting that next part. Some patients are looking to enhance athletic performance, and there are those who want to do better with the ladies - or the men. Many just want to remain competitive in the marketplace. Then there are those with challenging issues: they're tired and weak, they can't think or sleep, or they've lost their sex drive. They're suffering perhaps from a spectrum of issues and they're motivated to change.

Here's what I tell them, "You can do it the old way, or you can do it the new way. Either way will be difficult." Lifestyle change means breaking old habits and forming new ones, which is one of the hardest things a human can do. I respect that and try not to overwhelm people. I pick the low hanging fruit as best as I can, and don't tackle every problem immediately, but there has to be a basic level of motivation to start with. In order to help, I need to understand why they have come to see me and what they are capable of doing for themselves.

Like all things in life, some people can handle change better than others. What I've learned is that if people truly commit themselves and take small, manageable steps, they can achieve truly remarkable results.

GET WITH THE PROGRAM

CHAPTER 3

For the practice of anti-aging, the name of the game is change. As with all change, it's about understanding where you came from, where you are now, and where you want to go. The object is to modify your habits, behavior, and body chemistry. Doing so will enable you to come close to your true essence - which is an optimal, healthy, fully functioning human being.

So much of what we do in anti-aging relates to common sense and intuitiveness. Once we understand the principles and begin to practice them, it all seems natural. We must respect human biology. We often think we can ignore the basics, and in many ways, advanced technology does let us override the basic constraints faced by our ancestors; but we now

http://www.youtube.com/watch?v=dvla9 yV yI0

ignore how we have been biologically designed, and this is to our peril. If you disrespect your biological system, you pay a huge price. You will age faster.

A lot of anti-aging is about understanding your body, and giving it the respect it deserves. When you achieve this, it will respect you back and you'll live longer, feel better, and achieve your goals of health, energy, and youthfulness.

Most of the disrespect we have for our basic biology is due to lack of knowledge. Basically, people do what they know, which generally means what they've been told and what they've learned, even if the information is incorrect. They just don't know any better, and unfortunately, in the course of picking up that information, they've formed bad habits.

As an anti-aging physician I am constantly faced with people doing things based on false or inaccurate information. Many of my patients have formed habits that are detrimental, and extremely difficult to break. That is the challenge I face with each patient.

THE BASICS

The perspective we need is pre-technological. Think back ten thousand years, before civilization but after the millions of years it took to evolve the human form. Did we have electric lighting then? No. Did we have transportation machinery then? No. Did we have air conditioning? No.

In those very early days, humans slept when it was dark, got exercise from daily travels, and broke into a sweat at least once every day. People today have lost track of that. Modern conveniences have made life easier, which is a good thing, but in some ways have made many of us unintentionally lazy, which is not good. We think our biology has suddenly been reinvented because of technology, but it hasn't. Our bodies are still the same, but advancements in technology have interfered with our ability to understand and respect our biological needs. Our behavior has changed for the worse, which is why we have to change our behavior to pursue anti-aging.

Before you resist the idea of changing yourself, let me remove the red flag. The changes you are going to make in order to become more youthful are gradual. Improvement is a step-by-step process, and you will find with health that small incremental improvements can have exponential benefits. This is not widely understood, but it is true. You don't have to reach your goal weight to feel positive effects of weight loss; if you lose fifteen or twenty pounds, the health benefits are huge.

Our objective with RVI patients is not only getting people to reach their ideal. Of course you try, but there are obstacles to reaching that ideal, most of which have to do with the patients themselves. It's not that it can't be done, but I have found that it is hard for most people to do everything I want them to do. If I get too tough on people I will lose them, and I don't want to lose them because I want to help them.

In the practice of holistic anti-aging, there is a fine line between doing everything that needs to be done and doing enough to achieve improvements that can be seen, felt, and appreciated. That is part of the art of anti-aging medicine; always moving in the right direction. This goes for doctors as well as patients. If you see a doctor who is an advocate of anti-aging, but looks like he/she is not following their own message, they aren't going to have a lot of credibility.

So, how do we get there, to a life of vigor, energy, youthfulness, mental keenness and physical stamina? Overall we need to look at anti-aging within the context of wellness, and that means cleaning up the environment we live in.

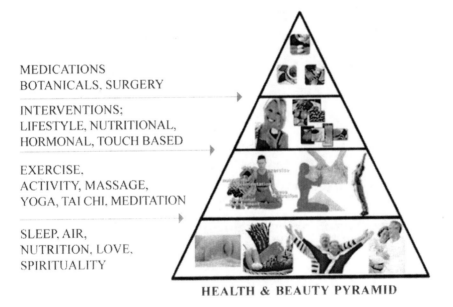

MEDICATIONS
BOTANICALS, SURGERY

INTERVENTIONS;
LIFESTYLE, NUTRITIONAL,
HORMONAL, TOUCH BASED

EXERCISE,
ACTIVITY, MASSAGE,
YOGA, TAI CHI, MEDITATION

SLEEP, AIR,
NUTRITION, LOVE,
SPIRITUALITY

HEALTH & BEAUTY PYRAMID

THE MODEL

We need to look at wellness as that strong and balanced table mentioned earlier. That table is the foundation for anti-aging.

All of the more exotic or esoteric things we are going to look at, including hormone replacement therapy and neurotransmitter balance, simply won't work without a strong foundation. To recap, the foundation table has four legs: four pillars that support any anti-aging program. They are: **nutrition, exercise, sleep,** and **stress management**. If these four legs are solid, meaning you understand and apply our basic principles, then you've basically got the right lifestyle, and that's your foundation.

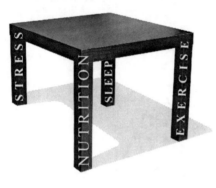

There are subtleties within each of these legs, of course, all kinds of little variations you can use in your approach to nutrition, exercise, sleep, or dealing with stress; but even the smallest lifestyle behaviors fall within these four main categories. Once they are under control and the legs of your foundation table are solid, then comes restoration and balance of your endocrine system a.k.a. your hormones, followed by your neurotransmitters. We are now going to look at each of the four anti-aging table legs in practical detail.

Let's get started with the program.

DIET AND NUTRITION

CHAPTER 4

I am often asked, "What is the most important thing someone can do to slow down or reverse the aging process?" Let's say this someone needs improvement in all four of our basic areas; that's clearly too much to take on at once, so we focus on the order of importance, and diet always comes first.

http://www.youtube com/watch?v=sv5- DQO3YY8

OUR DIETS ARE KILLING US

One great delusion of the modern age is that our diet has improved, and that we are living longer as a result. While it is true that a better diet has an impact on longevity, one of the great misperceptions today is that the average human lifespan has doubled in the last two hundred years because of diet. The only shred of truth to this lies in the historic context of mortality caused by starvation. Because of reduced starvation, our average lifespan has gotten longer, but the reality is that the biggest gains in increasing lifespan have come from hygiene and antibiotics, not from an improvement in our diets.

One of the great stories in medicine is that of Dr. Ignaz Semmelweis, a Hungarian obstetrician who discovered in the 1840s that infant mortality was greatly reduced if physicians washed their hands before delivering babies. His notion - that good hygiene can protect against infection and disease - was opposed by the medical establishment of his day, which believed that diseases were caused by "humours' in the body (the recommended treatment was bloodletting). Semmelweis was ostracized for his assertions, ultimately suffering a nervous breakdown and ending up in a mental asylum where he died, ironically enough, of an infection.

Despite the clinical evidence that it worked, it took thirty years for Semmelweis' idea to become accepted. Eventually his theory had a profound effect on both infant and adult mortality rates, as did the discovery of antibiotics, which helped reduce the huge epidemics that periodically cut short the lives of much of the population.

Great Truths

"All great truths goes through three stages:

• Ridicule
• Violently attacked
• Finally, accepted as self evident!"

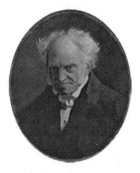

Arthur Schopenhauer
1788 - 1860

I like this story because it is an analogy for what happens in the advancement of science in general, and medicine in particular. Many ideas are opposed for no reason other than they go against the status quo. I see the same thing happening in anti-aging medicine. A great many commonly accepted ideas must be overturned, and new ways of doing things must be embraced. One of the incorrect yet commonly accepted ideas is that our diet as a nation, and as a species, has so improved that we are living longer as a consequence. Again, this is simply false, except in the context of starvation.

FOOD IS MEDICINE

I strongly believe that over time, food is more powerful than any pharmaceutical I could ever prescribe, but the concept that food is medicine is quite frequently lost in the aging equation. When

http://www.youtube.com/watch?v=roDJv6Bt8rQ

you understand it, you realize that most people are taking toxic doses of the wrong kind of medication at every meal. At the very least, they are receiving inadequate medication, because they're eating food that is low in nutrients.

The disturbing reality here is that we are facing a crisis of epidemic proportion when it comes to our diets.

Public Enemy #1: Poor Nutrition

The North American diet is greatly depleted of nutrition. We've leached so many naturally occurring vitamins and minerals from our soil, that our plants no longer get them and so can no longer pass them on to us. On top of that we process most of our food, so we destroy even more vitamins and minerals that way. We also add unnatural ingredients, either by exposing our foods to chemicals or by adding chemicals directly to them.

http://www.youtube.com/watch?v=6Qq W5DEqv0g

Fast food companies are downright criminal in this regard, if not from a legal point of view then surely from an ethical or moral perspective. They are certainly not doing anything to support anti-aging. Fast food is actually accelerating aging, illness, and obesity, and costing billions of dollars in taxpayer money to treat the consequences. Then consider the suffering people experience when they get sick, visit doctors, enter hospitals, and otherwise miss out on a healthy quality of life. All this hardship is caused by food.

The consequences of poor nutrition in America are endless and pathetic. Most Americans are clueless about what they eat. They listen to the food industry and shovel down whatever is marketed to them.

The Agro-Industrial Complex

When you go to a supermarket in America today, you find everything in the middle aisles handsomely boxed or packaged. People think they are getting all kinds of variety and wonderful selection, but most of it contains some form of processed corn, which is slowly killing everyone. Most of this food is also full of preservatives, artificial flavors, and chemicals; inherently toxic stuff that is also derived from corn. Our bodies are not designed to eat so much corn, not to mention its by-products. In short, the American food industry is poisoning its citizens, slowly killing more people than any terrorist could hope to.

If you don't think the government knows about this, you are being naive. It's also very difficult to stop, because it's about money. The food and agriculture industries are huge, and largely controlled by the same five or six mega-billion-dollar companies with a lobby as strong as the U.S. military.

I believe the agriculture industry has contributed enormously to disease and aging. We are all complicit, all part of a culture that has allowed this to happen. We believe that what we know about food we learned in school, or at home, or through traditions, but if you really examine what we learned about food from our schools, homes and traditions, it amounts to very little. What most of us know about food comes from paid advertisements run by companies that basically want to sell us junk.

A good example of this is the term 'corn-fed beef'. In the days of the Marlboro Man, that was the slogan for quality beef, but that was just the beef industry putting their spin on a cheaper way to produce meat. Who knew that grass-fed beef was so much better for you? This is exactly how people got educated about food, from the commercial conspiracy of big agriculture.

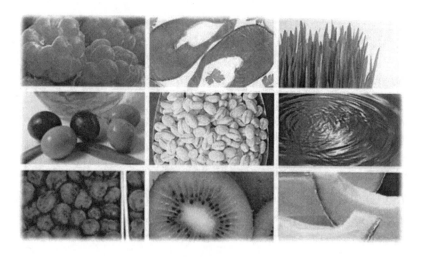

When I take food inventories of patients who come to my office, it is usually pathetic; both in terms of what people know, and what they eat. So I begin by giving them a few simple rules.

First, when you go into the supermarket, stay to the edge, the outside aisles. That is where the fresh, real food is. The stuff in the inner aisles is jammed with sugar, high-fructose corn syrup, and overly processed carbohydrates - offering little to no nutritional value. The second thing to keep in mind is: Buy organic food whenever possible.

There is a big difference between organic and non-organic food. Yes, organic costs more, but do you really want to put pesticides, antibiotics, and other artificial ingredients into your system? Artificial ingredients contribute to aging and chronic diseases.

ANTI-AGING SURVIVAL PROTOCOL
AIR Build your own air filtration box, place 1 or 2 units in each room in which you spend one-hour of time in or more
WATER Drink glass-bottled distilled water
SOIL Take a daily multivitamin/mineral supplement, preferably one that is vegetarian and free from artificial colors, preservatives, yeast, wheat, soy and milk
EMF De-technologize any room in your home in which you spend one-hour of time in or more - especially sleeping rooms
NUCLEAR RADIATION Know your risk - check how close you work and live to an active Nuclear Reactor, and be aware of emergency guidelines (http://www.nrc.gov/info-finder.html)
GMO FOODS Opt for locally grown, seasonally available fresh fruits and vegetables

FACTORS IN THE LIFE EXPECTANCY ROLLBACK

WATER POLLUTION & CONTAMINATION
- Babies born with 229 chemicals in their body; average NYC resident has 540 toxic chemicals in circulation
- Fish in 5 US rivers tainted with traces of prescription meditations: Lopid (never before found in wild fish); Zoloft; Prozac; Tegretol; Cardizem; others

AIR POLLUTION
- COPD (emphysema and chronic bronchitis) in the US: Is NOW the 3rd leading cause of death… Was 4th leading cause in 2002… Was 5th leading cause in 1990s

SOIL DEPLETION
- US farmland is over 85% micronutrient depleted
- Nutrient loss in potatoes over the last 50 years: 100% loss of Vitamin A; 57% loss of Vitamin C; 28% of Calcium; 50% of Riboflavin; 18% of Thiamine

LOW-DOSE EMF RADIATION
- NIH study (Feb. 2011) finds "evidence that the human brain is sensitive to the effect of RF-EMFs from the acute cell phone expocures"
- Argentinean team (Dec. 2011) reports that wi-fi singnals damage sperm

NUCLEAR RADIATION
- Fucushima Dai-ichi plant: radioactive core inside Reactor 1 burned through a concrete containment barrier and nearly reached the soil below; radiation - contaminated beef, vegtables, mushrooms found at markets 200 miles from the plant

GMO FOODS
- Soy, corn, canola, cotton and sugar beets have bacterical genes inserted; corn and cotton have a genetically-inserted pesticide
- In 2011 42% of the total arable land on Earth was planted with GM crops
- 80+% of the foods soils in supermarkets is GMO

HOW TO INCORPORATE
MORE ORGANIC FOOD INTO YOUR DIET

Most of my patients are not preparing meals just for themselves, but also for a spouse/partner and children. In order for dietary changes to become a successful part of your lifestyle, it's important that your entire household both supports you and actively participates. In my practice, I have found the following to be incredibly helpful when making the transition to organic shopping, cooking and eating:

1. First of all, organic doesn't have to be purchased at the local health food store. Most cities (even large ones like Los Angeles) have regular, year-round farmers' markets. Make the market a part of your regular routine. Sometimes they're at lunchtime in downtown areas, and others are on weekend mornings in your neighborhood. Schedule your shopping visits and you'll find it's easier to go.

The vendors at these markets bring in produce that's grown locally. Not all of it is organic, but much of it is - just ask. It's interesting to see fruits and vegetables presented seasonally, and you'll find that not only is it fun to try new things, but prices can be very low for produce in season; in fact, often much lower than you find in the supermarket, since local vendors cut out the middleman. Many even offer free samples, which is a great way to try new foods. Some markets will also bring in other organic products such as honey, eggs, and meat, at prices well below what you'd pay at the supermarket.

If you cook with or for others, begin to engage them as well. Children are much more receptive to change when they're involved. Let your children help choose the produce. Talk about its health benefits. For younger ones, keep it simple with terms such as, "Oranges have vitamin C. That helps your body fight off nasty colds." Don't be discouraged if your family is resistant. You're asking them to change a lifetime of bad habits, too.

2. The second thing you can do is consider planting a small garden. Obviously, space can be a concern, but you don't need much and you can start off slowly. Lettuce and other greens grow quickly if they're not in direct sun all day, and can actually grow year-round in some climates.

Tomatoes need good sunlight to ripen fully, but most climates get at least a few weeks of strong sunlight each year. If you're timid about gardening or less committed to growing a green thumb, start off with a couple of containers. You'll be surprised what a few seeds, some water and sunlight, and a little elbow grease can yield; and there's nothing more rewarding than eating a meal prepared with fresh ingredients from your own garden.

You might say, "Dr. Berger, I eat fast food and processed foods, and they haven't killed me!" This is because nutritional and agricultural toxins act incrementally, slowly, and silently. They contribute to silent inflammation, a fundamental cause of poor health and aging, and their effects may not manifest for decades.

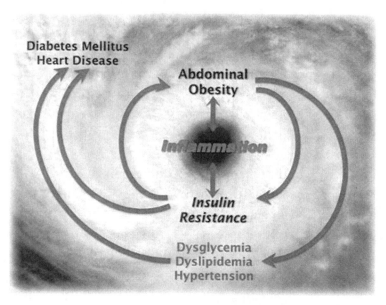

The Perfect Storm - Obesity & Inflammation

Remember that morning you looked in the mirror and thought, "Did I age overnight?" It has actually developed over the years without your awareness. You're living your happy life, doing your happy things, feeling relatively well, and then, all of a sudden, you have a heart attack, or your memory starts to go. The diseases associated with aging start years earlier, and silently develop until your body can no longer cope with the onslaught of poor nutrition, and diseases begin to express themselves. Food is something you actually put in your body and have control over. Make sure it's pure.

Less Is More

Once my patients understand that quality is essential, we address quantity. One of the main things I look at is calories. The reality is that most people in the United States consume too many and are overweight. Even in Southern California, the mecca of health and fitness and the place where I practice anti-aging medicine, about half of my new patients are overweight. In the rest of the country it's probably sixty-five to seventy percent.

OBESITY TRENDS* AMONG U.S. ADULTS

BRFSS 2009
(*BMI ≥30%, or ~ 30 lbs. overweight for 5' 4" person)

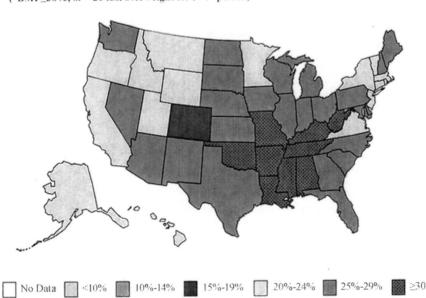

No Data   <10%   10%-14%   15%-19%   20%-24%   25%-29%   ≥30%

In my evaluation, I closely look at each patient's body composition. I measure weight, height, percentage of body fat, percentage of lean muscle mass, and what their percentage of water is. If they have an abnormal body composition, it's either that they have too much fat, too much fat and too little muscle, or they are okay with fat but have too little muscle (sometimes there is a case of too much fat and too much muscle, but that is rare).

Progress to Type 2 Diabetes

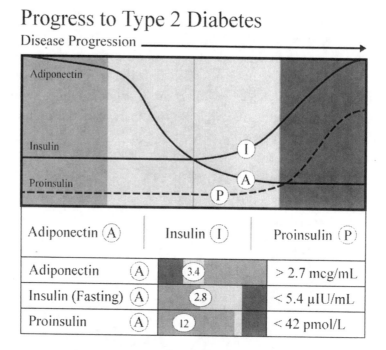

Adiponectin (A)	Insulin (I)	Proinsulin (P)
Adiponectin (A)	3.4	> 2.7 mcg/mL
Insulin (Fasting) (A)	2.8	< 5.4 μIU/mL
Proinsulin (A)	12	< 42 pmol/L

While some of the problem relates to the kinds of food they eat, equally important is the discussion about how much food they eat; we need to talk about portion size and calories. People need to achieve normal muscle mass and a normal percentage of body fat - i.e. a more balanced body composition - which has a direct relationship to health and wellness. It's a fairly simple deal. Body weight stays stable as long as the number of calories consumed equals the number expended from physical activities and metabolic processes. If you take in more calories than you need, the excess is used to build new tissue, especially fat, and you are going to gain weight. This is something that typically happens more when you get older, for a variety of reasons. On the other hand, the reverse occurs if you take in fewer calories than you need: Body size reduces and you experience subnormal weight. This may be a problem because in most cases it means a loss of lean muscle mass.

The reason most patients are not very successful with weight loss when left to their own devices, is that weight loss is self-limiting. As we lose weight and our bodies shrink in size, the amount of food needed to move and maintain our body mass shifts to a new, slower plateau consistent with the new weight. The initial weight loss causes changes in hormones, the autonomic nervous system and the built-in efficiency of muscle that collectively serves to protect us and conserve energy. It then becomes way more difficult to lose more weight, requiring even more calorie restriction and more rigorous physical activity. Unfortunately, most people do exactly the opposite after losing weight; they go back to their original diet and exercise habits and predictably regain the pounds. I am often able to help patients work through these plateaus and get back on track with their weight loss goals.

Staying Strong

One of the important things I let my overweight patients know is that the body, per se, doesn't differentiate easily between types of calories. If you are on a diet and all you think about is restricting calories, not thinking about the types of calories, you are going to lose muscle along with fat. People think, "I'm going to lose this weight and it's all going to be fat," but in fact it's going to be fifteen to twenty percent muscle loss. That is not good. The ideal way to approach your goal weight, if you in fact need to lose weight, is to lose fat and preserve muscle mass, so the first thing patients need is an adequate amount of protein, the stuff that muscle is made from. Anything less than the minimum amount, which I will discuss, means a high risk of losing muscle mass along with fat.

THE ANTI-AGING DIET

A "New" Therapeutic Approach to the Treatment of Malignant Brain Karkinos

"Let Food be your Medicine and Medicine be your Food"

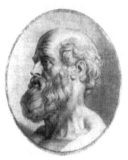

Hippocrates
460 BC - 370 BC

The diet I prescribe is quite a bit different from the one you may have seen in school on the food pyramid. Those diets contain too many refined carbohydrates, for a start, plus they have you eating too much of the wrong things and too little of the right. A healthy diet includes organic sources of lean protein, natural carbohydrates, healthy fats, and the elimination of any foods that cause sensitivities.

At RVI I prescribe a diet customized to each patient's unique situation. I consider their metabolism, acquired habits, and their ability to consistently improve their eating choices and remain disciplined and committed to following their new nutritional regimen.

Protein sources should be lean with low levels of saturated fat. Carbohydrates should primarily come from vegetables (eighty percent) with the rest from fruit, legumes, and whole grains. Saturated fats should be limited to less than eleven percent of total calories.

http://www.youtube.com/watch?v=Z3sP67CvY-I&feature=youtu.be

I determine the ideal total daily calorie intake by performing metabolic testing and referencing the patient's resting energy expenditure - which is essentially the amount of calories they burn at rest. I then adjust this number to take into account the patient's body composition and activity level. The ultimate goal of the diet is to achieve an ideal body composition, or at least come as close as possible.

There is one basic truth to weight loss: You need to burn more than you eat. Target Metabolic Zones tell you exactly how to do that. The following results of your test show you precisely how many calories your body actually burns, and calculates how many calories you should eat to lose or maintain your weight.

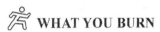

WHAT YOU BURN

HOW MUCH YOU EAT

EXERCISE + 145 Cals
(Estimated from Measurement)

This is an estimate of the number of Calories you would burn with 30 minutes at a moderate exercise level.

NEED TO BURN MORE CALORIES THAN YOU EAT!

LIFESTYLE
& ACTIVITY + 417 Cals
(Estimated from Measurement)

This is the number of calories you burn performing your daily activities... working, playing, eating, etc. Activities accounts for a significant portion of the Calories you burn each day.

MAINTENANCE ZONE
1397 to 1814

Once you reach your goal weight, this is how many calories your body needs to maintain your weight.

WEIGHT LOSS ZONE
1119 to 1397

Comfortable weight loss comes from eating slightly less Calories than your body needs. By eating healthy food throughout the day you should not feel hungry.

REE

RESTING ENERGY
EXPENDITURE
+ 1397 Cals
(Metabolic Measurement)

Today we measured your Metabolic Rate. This is the number of the Calories your body burns everyday at rests.

MEDICALLY SUPERVISED
ZONE - 0 to 1119
Medically Supervised Only

Very low calorie diets should only be done under medical supervision. Supervision is required to ensure adequate nutrition, and to monitor and treat the potential slowing of metabolic rate.

**CALORIES/DAY
1959 CALS*
TOTAL ENERGY OUTPUT**

CALORIES / DAY ENERGY INPUT

*TOTAL =REE + LIFESTYLE+ EXERCISE

How does your metabolism compare?
Compared to a typical person of similar sex, age, height and weight is:

SLOW   NORMAL   FAST

CAUTION: If you think you may not have sealed your nose or mouth around mouthpiece, or if you exercised or ate a large meal beforehand, you may want to repeat the test (ask about correct test preparation)
*note: NORMAL is considered to be +/- 10% the predicted value.

Once we have our goals set, I then introduce my patient to the RVI nutritionist. Using my prescription, the nutritionist translates my recommendations into a diet for everyday eating. This diet is very precise and broken down by the number of grams and percentages of carbohydrates, protein, and fat that must be consumed each day. This also includes a customized meal plan broken down into meals and snacks.

Protein

Most people eat too little or too much protein, or not the right proteins to fuel their body but you do need a minimum amount of protein to preserve muscle mass.

PROTEINS	CARBOHYDRATES	FATS
Necessary for maintaining youthful muscle mass. All cells have proteins, but primarily, dietary protein is necessary for maintaining adequate youthful muscle mass.	Necessary for short term energy. If you don't burn off the carbs that you need for energy production, you'll end up storing them as fat.	Fats are necessary for energy production and also for normal cell function. These are good fats, not bad fats. Bad fats are not necesarry at all and are a primary source of cellular inflammation. Overindulgence contributes to less than optimal aging and to development of chronic disease.
All of these are essential ingredients to optimal nutrition, however, it is about the quanitity that will determine how much they contribute to optimal wellness.		

What amount is the right amount? Right now we think we know what that number is, and have a formula. Basically you need about 1.5 milligrams of protein per kilogram of body weight (you divide your body weight in pounds by 2.2) on a daily basis. That's usually going to come to between 80 and 200 grams of protein a day, or about 1/4 pound to 1/2 pound. It's a simple calculation, and depends on your body weight. You need this minimum amount to preserve your lean body mass. In any given meal, a normal protein serving should be no more than three or four ounces of lean protein. That's adequate. In other words, eat a quarter pounder - just not a McDonald's Quarter Pounder.

If you have a normal body composition, you only need this much. If you want more muscle mass for whatever reason - if you want to improve your physique, for example - you need a little more. To maintain a constant level, 80-200 grams a day is how much protein you need; and yes, you can eat too much protein, but the consequences aren't nearly as bad as eating too many processed carbohydrates.

SAMPLE LIFESTYLE THERAPY PLAN

Sample Diet & Nutrition Rx and Edu

DIET AND NUTRITION: CUSTOM MEAL PLAN INSTRUCTIONS

Below is your prescribed breakdown of daily caloric intake.
As discussed, ideally your sources of carbohydrate, protein and fat should be from organic whole foods and not from processed foods.

PROTEIN:	SATURATED FATS:	CARBOHYDRATES:
Protein sources should be lean with low levels of saturated fat.	Saturated fats should be limited to less than 11% of total calories.	Carbohydrates should be primarily from vegetables equal to 80% and fruit and legumes 20%.

CUSTOM MEAL PLAN: PART 1		CUSTOM MEAL PLAN: PART 2	
CARBOHYDRATE 150gm 30%		Meal 1: 550 Kcal	Snack 1: 150 Kcal
PROTEIN 200gm 40%		Meal 2: 550 Kcal	Snack 2: 150 Kcal
FAT 67gm 30%		Meal 3: 450 Kcal	Snack 3: 150 Kcal
		TOTAL: 2000 Kcal	

The type and source of protein you ingest is very important. Most people know that low-fat protein - fish, seafood, lean meat, skinless poultry, etc. - is superior to fatty meats. Like other foods, organic is better. In the case of beef, organic means avoiding the chemicals pumped into cattle to fatten them up. In the case of chicken, it means cage free, as well as avoiding chemicals. If you can find it, eat grass-fed beef or bison. Those are magic words: grass-fed. You don't want something with recombinant bovine growth hormone (rBGH) in there, and you don't want something that is corn fed. You want your food eating the foods they were designed to eat.

Another great source of protein is eggs. The only contraindication to eggs is if you have a sensitivity or allergy to them. I don't think that eggs are even a contraindication for people with high cholesterol, because I don't believe it really matters. I explain why below.

Carbohydrates

Once we have established protein requirements, the next thing I calculate is whether the patient needs to be on a low carbohydrate diet or a very low carbohydrate diet. I do this by looking at the degree of insulin resistance they have, with a three hour or four hour glucose tolerance test with insulin. (See the section on sugar, insulin resistance, and diabetes in Appendix Two for more information.)

If they have an abnormal response, with either too much insulin or not enough insulin because of their resistance (or they are a little bit burned out as far as their pancreas is concerned), I put these patients on a very low carbohydrate diet. It's an Atkins-like approach, with fifty grams or less of carbs per day, which is pretty low.

If their response is closer to normal, I will put them on a low carbohydrate diet, which is anything less than 150 grams. This is still relatively low, because the average American diet has 350 grams of carbohydrates per day or more. I also explain the types of carbs that are optimal, because a low carb diet that is full of processed grains isn't providing your body with the nourishment and energy benefits we are seeking.

In terms of how this translates into basic food energy, the formula is simple. One gram of carbohydrate is equal to four calories, one gram of protein equals four calories, and one gram of fat equals nine calories. You can see that fat is denser in calories than protein or carbohydrates, so you need less of it.

Fats

When doctors talk about reducing fat, most of them are hoping to reduce fats to reduce cholesterol. Most of the time, a low carbohydrate diet alone, with whole-food carbohydrates, will immediately lower triglycerides and LDL cholesterol and raise HDL cholesterol.

What we really need to focus on is a reduction in saturated (animal) fat, and I like to bring my patients down to less than eleven percent total saturated fat. On the other hand, everyone needs adequate good fat, which is actually beneficial. This includes omega-3 fatty acids, fish oil, and mono-unsaturated fats such as olive oil, canola oil, safflower oil, and coconut oil. These are all fine, and will improve your cholesterol numbers. Other food sources of good fat include avocado and nuts. I tell all of my patients to eat some nuts, have some avocado, have some fish, and take some extra fish oil.

The Big C (Cholesterol)

Based on my experience, and a great deal of research, I believe the whole traditional notion of cholesterol is wrong. High cholesterol really isn't the problem. The problem is oxidized, low-density cholesterol: the low-density lipoprotein (LDL) cholesterol and the very low-density lipoprotein (VLDL) cholesterol in particular. Total cholesterol, by comparison, is almost a meaningless number.

What gets us into trouble is the oxidation of the cholesterol particle, not the total cholesterol number. If you break down the cholesterol panel you have high-density lipoprotein, or HDL, which is the good cholesterol, and low-density lipoprotein, or LDL, which is the bad cholesterol because it gets oxidized. There is also the very low-density VLDL cholesterol that is an even smaller particle than LDL and also gets oxidized.

These oxidized, low-density lipoproteins are instrumental in coronary artery plaque formation via the silent inflammatory process. It is this silent inflammation that causes many of the illnesses we associate with old age such as heart disease, cancer and dementia. In the case of heart disease, it's inflammation through the oxidation of these low-density and very low cholesterol particles that is the cause. It has little to do with total cholesterol per se.

You need a certain amount of cholesterol in order to make adequate amounts of sex and adrenal hormones; for example, if your cholesterol gets too low you can't make enough testosterone. That is one of the big problems with statins and other drugs that knock down cholesterol levels; patients on these drugs often come in with a testosterone deficiency, or adrenal fatigue with low cortisol. So, cholesterol isn't an issue as much as the oxidation of LDL and VLDL cholesterol.

As for the kinds of proteins, carbohydrates, and fats you should eat, that can become a long list, and endless diet books have been written on the subject. I do not tell my patients what specifically to eat - since everyone has their own likes and dislikes - but I do indicate the amounts and percentages of protein, carbs, and fats that should be eaten, based on my assessments of each patient as outlined above. Depending on their existing diet, they may also need to greatly reduce or eliminate certain foods.

Two things you can always be sure of:

1) I tell patients to stop eating processed foods and eat organic as much as possible.

2) Food is medicine, and you do not want to be eating or drinking food that has been degraded or has pathogens or toxins.

OBSTACLES TO PROGRESS: FOOD SENSITIVITY

One obstacle to the new diet may be food sensitivities. Food sensitivities can cause a range of symptoms, from gas and bloating to skin disorders such as eczema and psoriasis, to headaches and lethargy. Obviously, these symptoms don't mesh well with our plan to create a newly revitalized patient.

I generally test my patients for sensitivities to about two hundred foods, using a basic food sensitivity test. Some sensitivities are severe - causing a significant reaction - while others are much weaker. Some foods must be eliminated permanently, while others need to be eliminated for only six months, and then we can try reintroducing them. There's another list of weaker sensitivities they can rotate through; these foods should be eaten no more than every four days or so.

If a patient doesn't want to do a food sensitivity test, I'll eliminate certain basic problematic foods, such as dairy products. Up to ten percent of the population is sensitive to the lactose in dairy products, so that's an obvious first step. Dairy may also contain casein and whey, which a lot of people have problems with. You may not want to eliminate those foods, but you should really try to reduce them. If you want yogurt I recommend unsweetened Greek-style yogurt, which has some beneficial bacterial cultures. It's good for gastrointestinal health, as long as you don't have a sensitivity or allergy. If you're going to drink milk, drink non-fat organic milk.

Another way we can improve our health is to give up or cut down on foods that contain gluten, a special kind of protein found in rye, wheat, and barley. In other words, you'll find gluten in most cereals and bread. It's what gives bread its chewiness, and what lets it soak things up. It's also associated with some fairly worthless carbohydrates, like white bread. Many people are sensitive to gluten. Fortunately, it's not found in grains that are really good for you, like oats and buckwheat.

FOOD SENSITIVITY TEST SAMPLE

SEVERE INTOLERANCE:
- Bass
- Numteg
- Cauliflower
- Orange
- Corn
- Plum

MODERATE INTOLERANCE:
- Buckwheat
- Cherry
- Chick Pea
- Chicken
- Flaxseed
- Ginger
- Mushroom

MILD INTOLERANCE:
- Anchovy
- Cayenne Pepper
- Duck
- Leek
- Avocado
- Cocoa
- Egg Yolk
- Lime
- Beet
- Crab
- Goat's Milk
- Sesame
- Cashew
- Cranberry
- Lamb
- Walnut

ACCEPTABLE FOODS

VEGETABLES:
- Acorn Squash
- Broccoli
- Celery
- Green Pepper
- Kidney Bean
- Mustard
- Pinto Bean
- Soybean
- Sweet Potato
- White Potato
- Artichoke
- Brussel Sprouts
- Cucumber
- Iceberg Lettuce
- Lentil Bean
- Navy Bean
- Radish
- Spinach
- Swiss Chard
- Zucchini
- Asparagus
- Cabbage
- Eggplant
- Jalapeno Pepper
- Lima Bean
- Okra
- Rhubarb
- Squash (Yellow)
- Tomato
- Black-eyed Pea
- Carrot
- Green Pea
- Kale
- Mung Bean
- Onion
- Romanie lettuce
- String Bean
- Turnip

FRUIT:
- Apple
- Blueberry
- Grape
- Lemon
- Papaya
- Pomegranate
- Watermelon
- Appricot
- Cantalope
- Grapefruit
- Mango
- Peach
- Pumpkin
- Banana
- Date
- Honeydew (Melon)
- Nectarine
- Pear
- Raspberry
- Blackberry
- Fig
- Kiwi
- Olive
- Pineapple
- Strawberry

MEAT:
- Beef
- Turkey
- Liver
- Veal
- Pheasant
- Venison
- Pork

DAIRY:
- Cows Milk
- Egg White
- Sheep Milk

SEAFOOD:

- Clam
- Halibut
- Salmon
- Snapper
- Tuna

- Coofish
- Herring
- Sardine
- Sole
- Whitefish

- Crayfish
- Lobster
- Scallop
- Swordfish

- Haddock
- Oyster
- Shrimp
- Trout

GRAINS:

- Millet
- Rice
- Tapioca

HERBS/SPICES

- Basil
- Cinnamon
- Mint
- Sage

- Bay Leaf
- Clove
- Oregano
- Tarragon

- Black Pepper
- Cumin
- Paprika
- Thyme

- Chili Pepper
- Dill
- Parsley
- Tumeric

NUTS/ OILS AND MISC. FOODS:

- Almond
- Brasil Nut
- Carob
- Fructose
- Hops
- Pecan
- Sunflower

- Baker's Yeast
- Brewer's Yeast
- Coconut
- Garlic
- Macadamia
- Pistachio
- Vanilla

- Beet Sugar
- Cane Sugar
- Coffee
- Hazelnut
- Maple Sugar
- Psyllium
- Black Tea

- Green Tea
- Caraway
- Cottonseed
- Honey
- Peanut
- Safflower

CANDIDA

YOU HAVE NO REACTION TO CANDIDA ALBICANS.

GLUTEN/GLIADIN

YOU HAVE NO REACTION TO GLIADIN AND MODERATE REACTION TO GLUTEN, AVOID THESE FOODS:
- Barley
- Malt
- Oat
- Rye
- Wheat

CASEIN/WHEY

YOU HAVE NO REACTION TO CASEIN OR WHEY.

Sugars

For the elimination list I prefer to use something called the glycemic load. As discussed in the section on carbohydrates, the glycemic load has to do with how fast the glucose from a particular food enters the blood stream, which determines how fast it raises your insulin level.

GLYCEMIC LOAD SAMPLE

FOOD	GI Value Glucose = 100	Nominal Serving Size	Available Carb per Serving	GL per Serving
All-Bran*. breakfast cereal	30	1/2 cup	15	4
All Sport ™ (orange) sports drink	53	8 oz	15	8
Almonds	[0]	1.75 oz	0	0
Angel food cake. 1 slice	67	1/12 cake	29	19
Apple, 1 medium	38 (avg)	4 oz	15	6
Apple, dried	29	9 rings	34	10
Apple juice. pure. unsweetened. reconstituted	40	8 oz	29	12
Apple muffin, small	44	3.5 oz	41	18
Apricots. fresh, 3 medium	57	4 oz	9	5
Apricots. canned in light syrup	64	4 halves	19	12
Apricots, dried	30	17 halves	27	8
Arborio, risotto rice, boiled	69	3/4 cup	53	36
Artichokes (Jerusalem)	[0]	1/2 cup	0	0
Avocado	[0]	1/4	0	0
Bagel, white	72	1/2	35	25
Baked beans	38 (avg)	2/3 cup	31	12
Baked beans, canned in tomato sauce	48 (avg)	2/3 cup	15	7
Banana, raw, 1 medium	52 (avg)	4 oz	24	12
Banana cake, 1 slice	47	1/8 cake	38	18
Barley, pearled, boiled	25 (avg)	1 cup	42	11
Basmati rice, white, boiled	58	1 cup	38	22
Beef	[0]	4 oz	0	0
Beets, canned	64	1/2 cup	7	5
Bengal gram dhal, chickpea	11	5 oz	36	4
Black bean soup	64	1 cup	27	17
Black beans, boiled	30	4/6 cup	23	7
Black-eyed peas. canned	42	2/3 cup	17	7
Blueberry muffin, small	59	3.5 oz	47	28
Bok choy, raw	[0]	1 cup	0	0
Bran Flakes™, breakfast cereal	74	1/2 cup	18	13
Bran muffin, small	60	3.5 oz	41	25
Brazil nuts	[0]	1.75 oz	0	0
Breton wheat crackers	67	6 crackers	14	10

Foods that have a lot of their sugar bound up in fiber have a lower load, and will release the sugar more slowly. These foods are better for you.

As we get older, high glycemic load foods have a greater impact on both weight and insulin. I tell patients to stick to whole food carbs that have a glycemic load of ten or less - oatmeal, for example, or beans. I give every patient a book that helps them keep track of the glycemic load in the foods they are thinking of eating or have eaten, to help guide them in their decisions.

A good example of a high fiber fruit with a low glycemic load is an apple. A good example of a low fiber fruit with a high glycemic load is a banana. Unless you happen to be tennis player Rafael Nadal, who eats a banana before he plays (probably for the potassium), I would cross banana off your list, but leave apple on it.

In the carbohydrate realm, generally pasta is better than a potato, which is better than rice, which is better than bread, which is better than breakfast cereals, which are for the most part processed from corn. Nothing beats protein in the form of fish, fowl or animal, since protein has a zero glycemic load - glycemic load only applies to carbohydrates.

Rethinking Carbs (or Vegetables Are Us)
The other food group with a negligible glycemic load is the green stuff.

Protein provides some energy, but it's primarily used for muscle building. It's not a significant source of energy unless you are on a very low carb diet. If you are on a very low carb diet, you will convert some protein and fat into energy otherwise more efficiently provided by carbs. We need carbohydrates as an efficient energy source.

This is really a Paleolithic-style diet. Remember that while it's important to get enough protein, it is more readily available today than it was to our ancestors. This is especially true of animal protein. They had to hunt for it, so they got a lot of their protein from vegetables and legumes. These foods can be very rich in proteins if you eat enough of them. Since they weren't always successful at fishing or hunting, their diets were rich in foods they gathered.

Today we have an abundance of everything. In the old days we didn't have refrigerators, we didn't have supermarkets, we couldn't preserve food and we really didn't process any. Just remember that while our diets have changed, our biology is the same. There are good carbohydrates and there are bad carbohydrates. Good carbohydrates should be the main staple of your diet. There's much to be said for vegetarianism, which is associated with longevity. That's because it's a low calorie diet and the carbohydrates vegetarians eat are mostly whole food carbohydrates that come from nature in the form of vegetables and fruits. A diet rich in vegetables is the ideal diet. Fill two-thirds of your plate with vegetables, and the other third with lean protein and possibly some whole grains or legumes. The more high-fiber phytonutrients you get from whole food carbohydrates, the better off you'll be.

Raw Please

So now you know the cardinal rule of healthy, anti-aging nutrition: your diet should be rich in vegetables and fruits. Our bodies desperately require an adequate and substantial amount of phytonutrients that vegetables and fruits provide - the more the merrier. These foods are also low in calories, high in fiber, and rich in nutritional value.

Generally speaking, vegetables and fruits are best when raw. Long cooking times and long storage times deplete their nutrients. (A big exception to this is the tomato, which releases the antioxidant lycopene when cooked.)

If you cook vegetables, less time is best. Have you ever noticed that when you cook a green vegetable in water, the water turns green? That green water you pour down the drain contains vital nutrients that your body is seeking. Steaming is better than boiling, because nothing much is leached out, and quick boiling is better than long stewing, for the same reason. I'm not saying we should consume raw foods exclusively, but they are the richest in nutrients. So, once again, aim to strike a balance.

REAL NUTRITION = REAL CHANGE

In the end, what we want is to 'clean up' the diet, to contribute to cleaning up our internal environment. It comes down to basic rules: eat whole, non-processed foods, and eat organic (including your meat) as much as possible. You should also get into the habit of reading food labels. You need to know what you put in your body.

Do these things and you will be surprised at what happens. Once I change a person's eating habits, I have begun to change their rate of aging, as well as their overall health. My patients can measure the benefits in myriad ways, with perhaps no bigger result than how great they feel. In a matter of weeks, someone who is barely functioning can get their life back and start feeling normal again, just by changing their diet. That's how powerful nutrition is.

EXERCISE

CHAPTER 5

Similar to the first pillar of our foundation, the second pillar, exercise, is best understood in terms of our Paleolithic lifestyle. This means examining how we lived for a millennium before the Neolithic Age of tools and technology, back when we were hunters and gatherers.

The problem is simple; we are woefully deficient in exercise. Our modern, Western style societies have become progressively more sedentary. We sit all day in a chair, moving little except for our mouths. Granted, people probably didn't have as much to say in the old days, and language was less evolved, but they moved. Today we get our exercise moving fingers across keyboards, picking up telephones, and turning steering wheels, but we are biologically designed to move. Our ancestors were big time movers; they had to be, to survive.

http://www.youtube.com/watch?v=qTaXnoDOQ7k

Very simply, we're designed to hunt and gather. For our ancestors, life was hard work; you had to go out every day and struggle. If you found food you were lucky. It was very time and energy consuming. Many hours each day were spent foraging, hunting, and preparing food. The body was in constant motion and the food they foraged was what fueled it.

We didn't have supermarkets, stores, or home delivery. We didn't have restaurants and drive-thrus. We just had our bodies and our wits. Now we've stopped moving, and that means we've stopped burning calories, which is just one downside to sedentary living.

THE OTHER BENEFITS OF EXERCISE

We all know exercise helps us maintain healthy body weight and composition, but there are other health benefits as well. Exercise combats the demineralization of bones, also known as osteoporosis.

It's bad enough to face the hormonal decline associated with aging, but if you haven't stimulated your bones by exercise, you're in trouble. You need to work your muscles because they are connected to your bones. Working muscles stimulates bones to mineralize; therefore exercise is essential for preserving the integrity of your bones.

Exercise also affects our brains in many positive, anti-aging ways. It releases stress. It improves blood flow in the body and the brain, improving cognitive function. Endorphins released during exercise make us feel better.

Hormonal balance is also improved by exercise, because of its effect on fat. Most people don't realize that fat is not a static piece of tissue; it is actually a very powerful endocrine organ. It secretes an amazing variety of hormones that influence our bodies in different ways. A sedentary lifestyle can affect fatty tissue in ways that cause hormonal disruption.

The relationship between exercise (or the lack of it) and fat (or an excess of it), contributes significantly to inflammation, the underlying cause of chronic diseases. Exercise and muscle mass are not just better from an aesthetic perspective, but also from a health, wellness, and anti-aging perspective. Too much fat equals too much inflammation, creating health problems down the line. Without exercise you can't have optimal body composition and all the health benefits that go along with that.

THE BEST EXERCISE FOR YOU

What are the best types of exercise? There is no best. Or better yet, the best kind of exercise is the kind you most enjoy doing - because you will actually do it. In terms of burning calories, however, exercise that creates more muscle will speed up your metabolism

http://www.youtube.com/watch?v=MG6wqtzPSW8

for a longer period of time. I always tell my patients that they need to mix up their exercise routine. You should do some aerobic exercises for immediate fat burning and for cardiovascular conditioning, but also do some muscle building and toning, because greater muscle mass will keep the engine idling at a higher RPM.

Muscle at rest burns calories, so building and maintaining it should be part of your exercise goal. I recommend doing interval type training; alternating lower intensity with higher intensity exercise within a defined heart rate range, so you can optimize both the cardiovascular as well as fat burning benefits.

Once you have these two basics down, you still have two more categories to satisfy: flexibility and balance. Some element of your exercise program should encompass these two essentials. Swimming, for example, is excellent for flexibility; fencing is great for balance; yoga is great for both.

Basically, for optimal results, you need to do some exercise in all four categories: fat burning cardio, muscle building, flexibility, and balance.

Fortunately, there are myriad ways of getting these exercises, and no single one is best for all categories. Within each category there are hundreds if not thousands of different exercises you can do. I recommend that my patients see our exercise physiologist or one of our affiliated trainers, who can help establish a custom designed program. However, anyone can craft their own routine, they just have to have fun, and they have to like it, because it has to be something they will want to keep doing every day.

As for frequency, when my patients ask, "How many days of the week should I exercise?" I say, "Well, how many days of the week are there? That's how many days you should exercise. If you want to take one day off, just don't lay in the bed that whole day, if you can help it." We are designed to move. Take one day off if you have to, but try to do something. Move every day.

This is looking at exercise in linear terms, of course, and mostly in terms of calories. Once we are past that, however, we are talking about maintaining a faster metabolism, a better cardiovascular system, and the more profound effects of exercise in terms of slowed or even reversed aging. The ultimate benefit comes down to very specific biological markers.

SAMPLE LIFESTYLE THERAPY PLAN		
Lifestyle therapy options: Exercise - Rx and Edu		

EXERCISE	TIME SUGGESTION	DAYS PER WEEK
1. Aerobic	20min (add 1 minute a day to reach 60 minutes)	6
2. Resistance	20min (add 1 minute a day to reach 60 minutes)	3
3. Stretching	Daily for 10 minutes after resistance or aerobic exercise	6
4. Balance	Daily for 10 minutes after resistance or aerobic exercise	6
5. Interval Trainnig	As much as possible for all exercise activities	1
6. With trainer		1

EXERCISE DETAILS	VALUE
Maximum heart rate = 220 - your age	170
70% max heart rate	119
85% max heart rate	145
1/2 way between 70% and 85%	132
Fat burning range (70% to 1/2 point)	119-132
Heart conditioning range (1/2 point to 85%)	133-145

The most significant study in recent years of the direct effect of exercise on aging was done in Germany in 2010. Results showed that serious middle-aged runners, people who ran fifty miles a week, had significantly longer telomeres than those of their contemporaries who did not exercise regularly. (Reminder: Telomeres are the end caps on our chromosomes that shorten over time until, in the end, the chromosomes unravel and the cell dies.) In other words, the anti-aging effects of regular exercise present on a cellular level.

To achieve this, you must find the best exercise for you, and that means finding the exercise that you are willing to commit to and actually do. That is the best exercise. You need this exercise for vitality, and to maintain weight, strength, flexibility and balance. These are all important things in order to feel strong and vital throughout your life. It's a core part of anti-aging.

GETTING STARTED

Exercise is vital. It's not an option. I tell my patients they have to exercise, they have to move. If they can, I want them to exercise every day. If they can manage an hour, that would be excellent, but any amount of exercise is far better than none at all. People don't realize the critical nature of getting at least some exercise; any movement will produce anti-aging and good health benefits.

Exercise is important on many levels, none more obvious than its importance in maintaining healthy weight. When you stop moving, you start storing fat, because you stop using the energy that you're taking in from calories. If you don't want to add fat, you must use up what you eat through exercise. It's simple. It's either eat and use calories, or eat and store fat.

Exercising regularly also increases your metabolic rate. This is critical because, astonishingly enough, you burn the majority of calories while resting. Your resting energy expenditure, determined by your basal metabolic rate, is by far most of what you burn. The amount you burn from exercise and activity is way less than what you burn doing nothing the rest of the day.

Weight is only one part of body composition. You want to maintain muscle tone and muscle mass as well, so you've got to use your muscles. Humans are not designed for sitting in a chair. I hate to think what we are going to look like in another fifty thousand years if we keep just sitting around.

In order to achieve and maintain your ideal body composition, I prescribe an exercise program for each of my patients, tailored to individual needs. For each patient we prescribe a combination of three types of exercise: cardiovascular conditioning, muscle training, and exercise for flexibility and balance.

1. Get Your Heart Pumping with Cardio

Cardiovascular workouts strengthen the heart and lungs. This is key to maintaining a healthy body composition. The goal is to start slowly and increase both intensity and frequency until you are doing moderately intense cardio at least thirty minutes a day, five days a week.

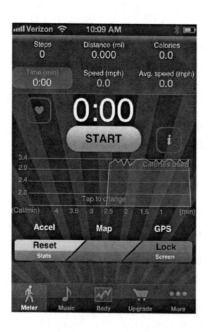

For patients who have never exercised before, we start off slowly and work our way up. While there are some people who don't like any form of exercise, most find one or two types more pleasurable than others, and I encourage patients to do what they like. Exercise doesn't have to be something you can only do at the gym. It can take the form of walking your dog, working in your garden, or finding a pickup basketball game at the park. It's all about moving, and then increasing the intensity to the heart rate zone right for you.

2. Keep Your Bones Healthy With Muscle Conditioning

Muscle conditioning, also called strength training, helps strengthen the muscles, bones, and connective tissue that support your body. It also is crucial for weight maintenance, as lean muscle raises your metabolic rate, which burns more calories.

Conditioning your muscles can be done in a variety of ways, from lifting barbell weights to using resistance bands, or engaging your own body's weight by practicing yoga. Many people assume that muscle conditioning is something that can be done less frequently as we age, but nothing could be further from the truth. Strength training is essential for improving bone density, which prevents us from breaking bones as we get older.

3. Stay Flexible and Balanced

You also need exercise for flexibility and balance. These are closely related and greatly affect how we react to and thrive in our physical environment. As you get older you lose your sense of balance, and any exercise you can do to maintain it is important. We must prevent balance-related problems such as falling, which can result in injury such as hip bone fractures.

Flexibility is closely related to balance. Flexibility involves being able to move our joints through their entire range of motion. While stretching isn't considered an exercise by many people, it's actually one of the most important exercises for keeping our bodies fluid, agile, and injury-free. Some types of exercise such as yoga and Pilates combine strength training, flexibility, and balance, and can be a good starting place for the exercise beginner or someone who is getting back to it after an extended period.

WHAT TO DO FIRST

There's no easier place to start than walking. It requires no special equipment, playing fields, (minimum time) limits, or other people. Walking is great for relaxation, and it may be the best exercise for some people, depending on their goals.

For best results, take at least fifteen to twenty thousand steps each day in order to burn enough calories. If you are only taking three or four thousand steps a day, you won't see much impact. To track your progress, I suggest getting a pedometer which counts how many steps you take. Everyone should have one. Then make sure you take enough steps daily. Twenty thousand steps is a lot for modern times, but that's what our ancestors did. They moved. And that's what we need do.

The sort of exercise program we design for ourselves, in the end, depends on our goals. For most people, the first goal is optimal body composition, which usually means losing weight while simultaneously building muscle mass. For this we want to create a caloric deficit. If you want to lose a pound a week, for instance, you have to have a 3,500 calorie deficit per week - an average of 500 calories per day; in other words, the equivalent of a McDonald's Quarter Pounder with cheese. Most people find it very difficult to create this calorie deficit without exercise.

Start Off Slowly

It's important to start your exercise program with something doable. Some patients are completely de-conditioned; they simply haven't been exercising. They are really out of shape, and can't begin with an hour of exercise every day. If I prescribed a program opening that intense, I would never see them again. I start most patients off slowly. First, I determine their maximum safe heart rate (220 minus their age). Then I calculate seventy and eighty-five percent of that heart rate for their individual target zone. I instruct them to exercise as much as possible using an interval method. For example, two minutes at a heart rate between seventy percent maximum and halfway between seventy and eighty-five percent. Following that, exercise for two minutes at a heart rate between eighty percent and eighty-five percent of maximum heart rate. Keep alternating between the high intensity and lower intensity in two minute intervals for the duration. I also recommend a quality heart rate monitor, so they can time themselves and monitor their heart rate simultaneously.

Depending on the case, I have even started patients with as little as ten minutes of moderate exercise daily. I tell them to add a minute each day, so in ten days, they are up to twenty minutes. In another forty days they are up to an hour, and they didn't even notice because it was a gradual progression they could easily accomplish.

One Day at a Time

Patients need to start exercising at a point where they can feel successful. This is crucial for motivation. It's the same with weight loss. I don't tell someone who needs to lose fifty pounds, "You need to lose fifty pounds!" We begin with, "You are going to lose five pounds," and after they lose the first five pounds, we discuss the next goal, and I assign the next five pounds, and so on. If I put a number like fifty in front of an already tired, frustrated patient, the reaction is, "Oh my god, I'll never be able to do that." I want people to focus on realistic goals that enable them to believe and push themselves into positive action. People come to me with hope, and my job is to make that hope work for them instead of against them. That's how we get the best results.

The same thing goes for exercise. If a patient takes on a tough program with a trainer and starts off working out several hours a day, they often are likely to quit. It's too much. On the other side of the coin are 'boot camp people'. They're motivated. They go to boot camp and work like crazy to get the weight off; but unless they pay serious attention to all the other long term lifestyle changes I've asked them to make, the weight starts creeping up as soon as boot camp is over.

There should be gradual, incremental increases in exercise. People who are already somewhat conditioned (working out three or four days a week, but still not reaching their goal), must increase their exercise level. Sometimes this is an hour's worth, sometimes two hours. Remember, it isn't only about time spent; a good hour of moderate exercise will only burn about five hundred calories. It's the resting energy expenditure that counts, and that may be very low, so we are looking to exercise in the best way to increase metabolism.

Of course, everybody is different. Some people are slow to change. while others are very motivated and don't want to wait a year to shed the extra weight. Those who exercise more lose weight faster. It's a very simple equation: calories in versus calories out.

EXERCISE

Current Exercise Program: Activity
(list type, number of sessions/week, and duration of activity)

Activity	Type	Frequency per week	Duration in Minutes
Stretching			
Cardio/Aerobics			
Strength			
Other (yoga, pilates, gyrotonics, etc.)			
Sports or Leisure Activities (golf, tennis, rollerblading, etc.)			

Rate your level of motivation for including exercise in your life: Low   Medium   High

List problems that limit activity:

Do you feel unusually fatigued after exercise?   Yes   No

If yes, please describe:

Do you usually sweat when exercising?   Yes   No

FITNESS OBSTACLES

Sometimes there are other obstacles to losing weight. challenges that keep your metabolism slow despite a healthy diet and exercise. While it sounds like a cliché when an overweight person blames their size on a hormonal imbalance problem. this can actually be the case.

If somebody is on a program of diet and exercise but not making the expected progress, we need to check for issues that can make it harder for fatty acids to leave the fat cells. We test for conditions like impaired thyroid function, high cortisol levels, low testosterone, low human growth hormone, or low progesterone. Hormonal imbalance can greatly impact weight loss. If you have a child who has subclinical hypothyroidism and eats a lot, he or she is going to put on weight faster than a child who has a fast metabolism and eats a lot.

Sometimes an overweight patient has other issues. If they are under stress, overeating can be a compensatory mechanism. Or there may a neurotransmitter imbalance in the brain - lower levels of gamma-amino butyric acid (GABA), or serotonin that result in a lack of sleep.

Lack of adequate sleep is a leading cause of obesity. Many adults and children have obstructive sleep apnea, which is a serious medical condition that causes lack of sleep and consequent weight gain, so is a big obstacle to successful weight loss. It must be diagnosed and treated.

There are many things that can contribute to excess weight. When it comes down to it, however, the most common contributing factors are poor diet and lack of exercise, which is why these are the first two steps we address in the RVI anti-aging equation.

SLEEP

CHAPTER 6

The problem we face is simple: very few of us get enough sleep. As a society, we suffer from sleep deprivation and sleep disorders in epidemic proportion. In order to get the desired results from the RVI anti-aging program, my patients need to get a sufficient amount of restful sleep on a regular basis.

http://www.youtube.com/watch?v=Zh-bB3p7fBc

HOW MUCH SLEEP DO YOU NEED?

It's become somewhat of a badge of courage in our culture, to brag about how little we sleep; and yet most adults need seven or eight hours of sleep per night to achieve the full restorative benefits. There are very few who can get by with less. There are some who think they can, but they are actually aging at an accelerated rate.

Your requirements for sleep change over time. In early adulthood you need more sleep, eight to ten hours. While that shifts down to the seven to eight needed during prime adulthood, as you age (in the traditional sense) you typically need more. We all hear of older people needing less sleep, but that's not exactly accurate. Many older people have sleep disorders, and hence, problems having a restful night.

HOURS OF SLEEP PER NIGHT BY AGE		
AGE	**HOURS**	Most beneficial time to sleep is when the sun is sleeping, in sync with natural rythms of light and darkness. Wake up with the sun. This is a natural rhythm. The more you deviate from that, the more you go against your natural physiology.
25 - 60	7 - 8	
60+	8 - 10	

Sleep disorders come in a variety of packages. Some are genetic. One patient of mine had a severe case of narcolepsy. Sufferers of this terrible genetic condition are prone to falling asleep suddenly and deeply, without notice or hesitation, at any time of the day. Without medication to keep her awake, she would fall asleep in the middle of a sentence. I mention this because it's the kind of thing people think of when you talk about sleep disorders. They think of it as something rare and strange, but sleep disorders are pervasive, as are the numerous causes for bad sleep - by which I mean an insufficient amount of restful sleep. The causes for bad sleep can be purely physical - obstructive sleep apnea, for example, a serious sleep disorder usually associated with obesity; or causes can be purely behavioral - sleep deprivation self-induced by a person's work or play habits. Then there is stress, which plays havoc with any sleep pattern.

Regardless of cause, the result is that too many people experience excessive daytime sleepiness, a clear sign of insufficient restful sleep. This is extremely harmful. The importance of sleep is something I cannot emphasize enough. If you take no other message from this book, take this: you will never be well until you sleep enough. You can achieve everything else - good nutrition, good exercise, and proper hormone balance - but if you don't get enough good sleep, you won't be healthy. It's like having three legs on a four-legged table. You have to sleep restfully, or the whole thing falls over.

We can't cut back on sleep, because too many critical physiological processes take place during the sleep cycle. Just because you're sleeping doesn't mean your body is. Your body not only restores itself during restful sleep, but repairs damage on the cellular level, something we refer to as immune surveillance. Your hormones are at work while you sleep. Growth hormone, for example, is only produced during sleep. When people are deprived of sleep, growth hormone levels go down, along with other hormones. Your pituitary gland function is particularly affected by sleep disorders.

For my patients, understanding that good sleep is key to anti-aging is part of their core education. We ask them extensively about their sleep patterns, test them for excessive daytime sleepiness, and counsel them on how to get better sleep. The message is, if you want to live longer, sleep more. Not too much, but enough.

The Night Shift

Another modern invention that is good for industry, but not so good for our health, is the night shift. People who work night shifts suffer because they are going against the grain of their normal biological rhythm. In addition, people who work the night shift come home when it is daylight and their internal clock is telling them to stay up and they try to squeeze in a few more hours of daylight before they go to sleep. This natural response to the night shift also causes sleep deprivation.

So, if at all possible, avoid the night shift. It will age you very quickly. Remember, before Thomas Edison ruined our ancient rhythms of sleep it was light, then dark, light, then dark, and so on.
Try to respect that.

THE IMPORTANCE OF BEING RESTED

The healing power of sleep has been part of our common wisdom for a long time, but interestingly enough, mainstream medicine has been slow to recognize this. Among other things, the medical profession is notorious for the long, sleepless hours of the medical residency that is part of every MD's training. It's like a fraternity hazing, a rite of passage.

The medical profession now wants to change this traditional passage of sleepless residencies for young doctors, largely because of what it does to their judgment, concentration, memory, and all the normal functions you expect and must count on a doctor to perform properly. The medical establishment has realized that you need seven or eight

http://www.youtube.
com/watch?v=uMR
nj2GDQo4

hours of sleep on average, regardless of being an adult between the ages of nineteen and twenty, forty to fifty, or sixty-five to seventy.

Just as crucial as quantity of sleep is the quality of sleep - how restful your sleep is. The most important question to ask somebody when he or she wakes up, is, "Do you feel refreshed?" Does it take half an hour to an hour each morning to get yourself feeling like you're ready to face the world? The next question we must ask about quality of sleep is, "Do you experience excessive daytime sleepiness?" If you are sleepy during the day, you aren't getting enough quality, restful sleep.

So how can we help you improve both the amount and quality of your sleep? We first break down the problem into the behavioral vs. the biochemical. Some people don't sleep well because their lifestyle is not conducive to adequate, restful, and beneficial sleep. Others don't sleep well because of a physical problem, a chemical imbalance, or a genetic defect.

ESTABLISHING GOOD SLEEP HABITS

http://www.youtube.com/watch?v=0I6tdfzET8c

For most people the problem is not enough sleep, and they consequently suffer from some degree of sleep deprivation. In our society this is a serious problem. It is a behavioral problem, but still a sleep disorder. In terms of the deleterious behavior, however, it's usually pretty simple to understand; people simply don't put in the time. They go to bed late and wake up early, or they don't sleep through the whole night for any number of reasons, which we'll examine. So certain behaviors need to change.

The biggest problem is that most people don't plan for sleep. Just like our basic, natural biology, sleep gets very little respect. We override our natural instincts, and don't listen to what our bodies are telling us.

If you want to understand this, just replicate life before Thomas Edison. Take a camping trip and don't bring any candles. Give it a couple of days and watch how your sleep cycles change. Unless you have biochemical issues, or anxiety and stress that keep you awake, most likely your sleep time is going to lengthen dramatically.

Most people don't realize their deficiency in sleep is because of all the stimulation they experience; including work, work, and work. For most people, work doesn't end at five o'clock or even six o'clock anymore. Thanks to the desktop computer, the laptop, the cell phone, and now the iPad, people can stay connected twenty four hours a day and often continue working until they are exhausted.

AVOID THESE STIMULANTS	
1.	Loud noise such as: music, TV, traffic, arguments
2.	Bright lights
3.	Caffeine
4.	Alcohol
5.	Processed Carbohydrates
6.	Stimulant medications
7.	Recreational drugs
8.	Work
9.	Stressful news, TV
10.	Financial discussions
11.	Arguments

You see this all the time in our crazy society. People work too much. I'm not talking about painters or musicians who love their work. Art is a relaxing type of work. I'm taking about everybody else. When they work, it's not an expression of artistic talent, passion or love, it's strictly in response to pressure - economic pressure, political pressure, competitive pressure - and this is what drives the majority of the population. This is also a big reason why the majority of the population suffers from sleep disorders and sleep deprivation.

Sleep deprivation, you see, doesn't only come from staying up too late. It's also from repeatedly waking up in the middle of the night, a result of another disorder that causes sleep disturbance: stress. Stress will interrupt restful sleep. If you have stress and anxiety, you have too much stimulation, too much cortisol, too much adrenaline, too much norepinephrine - all of it floating around while you think about your day at the office, or what you have to do, or how the stock market did, or your spouse or your girlfriend or boyfriend. With all these things racing through your head, you are going to have a tough time not only falling asleep, but staying asleep for a truly restful night.

Sleep Aids

Many of my new patients come into the office revealing that they take either prescription or over-the-counter sleep aids. They have often begun taking them for the reasons outlined in this chapter: non-restorative sleep, trouble falling asleep, anxiety about sleeping too little, and waking at night. The problem with sleep aids is that they don't address the issue of why the person is not sleeping well and, thus, doesn't offer a solution - only a Band-Aid. While patients don't like giving up medications that they feel are working, if I can get them to trust me and follow the program, they are soon sleeping well on their own and feeling much better.

Plan for Sleep

I teach people to respect sleep by planning for it. First, figure out what time you need to wake up, and count back 8 hours. Then, figure out how long it takes you to actually fall asleep. Is it thirty minutes? Is it ten minutes? Add that on. That's when you should be getting into bed, ready to sleep, lights out.

You also have to behave in such a way that before you lie down, you avoid stimulation. You need to give yourself a couple of hours to de-stress, relax, and prepare yourself for that refreshing sleep mode. If you're working or stimulated right up until the time you lie down, it's going to take you more than a short interval to fall asleep. In many cases you may wake up, or find yourself having non-restful sleep, because the stress, the anxiety, and the associated hormones of stress and anxiety won't let you sleep well.

In my practice, we teach people to avoid work for two hours before they go to sleep. During those two hours they should avoid stimulation. Lower the lights, soften the noise, stay out of traffic; avoid the news, the stock market, arguments, or political commentary (if you are invested in any way). Do soothing, feel-good things that are relaxing.

SLEEP THERAPY INSTRUCTIONS
Get 7-8 hours of restful sleep per night.
Determine what time you need to get up and count back 7-8 hours and that is the time you need to be asleep.
No work for three hours prior to bedtime.
Avoid stimulation for three hours prior to bedtime.
No exercise other than relaxation exercises (nice walk) for three hours prior to bedtime.
Develop and maintain an evening relaxation ritual.
Avoid alcohol, caffeine or large meals within four hours of bedtime.

We recommend developing a nightly ritual that will help you relax. By now you should know what makes you feel calm and content. If you don't, then start experimenting. Light an aromatherapy candle, read a book or a favorite magazine, sit by a fire, play some soft music, sip of cup of tea, soak in a bath or hot tub. You can combine any or all of these for your own ideal winding down routine. These are just a few suggestions and may not be a fit for you, but you get the idea. The point is to build an evening ritual that will help prepare you for sleep by reducing stimulation and encouraging relaxation. For two hours prior to going to bed each night, give your brain and your spirit a chance to chill out, so your body will do the same and let you rest the way you're supposed to.

Also avoid alcohol, caffeine or any other stimulant for several hours before bed, because as many of us know, their effects will further decrease your quality of sleep.

Another helpful tip is not to eat any heavy meals for several hours before trying to sleep. You want to avoid gas, indigestion, or any of the distractions that heavy meals may bring you. Finish dinner a solid four hours before sleep. In fact, it is healthy to fast for twelve hours overnight, between the last meal at night and first meal the next morning, at least four days a week.

HOW YOUR DIET AFFECTS YOUR SLEEP

One thing we know is that caloric restriction and periodic fasting are more in step with our biochemistry than excessive eating. Remember that our ancestors often had long intervals between meals, far more often than we do today. So, if you have an eight p.m. dinner, don't have breakfast until eight a.m. the next day. That, in and of itself, replicates a partial fast, and you will feel the impact pretty quickly.

A lot of people are dietary insomniacs, meaning that their restless sleep is caused by what they eat before they go to bed. When you eat in the evening, make sure to eat more protein than carbohydrates, because protein will be more relaxing while carbohydrates are more energizing. Certain proteins such as milk or turkey also have L-tryptophan, which has a very calming effect, but if you eat too many carbohydrates in the evening your insulin rises; then as you go to sleep it starts to fall, and that can cause restless sleep. In these cases a little dietary manipulation can do wonders.

Naps

In Spain, it is a cultural phenomenon to dine very late and go to sleep even later. The reason why Spain is not an exhausted nation is because of the siesta. They break their sleep into two shifts and this works. In the United States it does not work, because we are a society that does not tolerate people who take a daytime snooze. This is unfortunate.

I believe in naps. Naps are fantastic! If you are tired your body is telling you something. Go take care of it. Naps are actually very natural to humans, especially in terms of the climate where they evolved. In many parts of the world mid-day is so hot that you can't do anything anyway. So you might as well just go find a shady spot and rest.

BRAIN CHEMISTRY AND SLEEP

Sometimes changing your behavior is not enough to create good sleep, and you must solve physiological or biological problems. One physiological (as distinct from behavioral) cause for an inability to sleep well can be hormonal imbalance. Menopausal women with basic estrogen and progesterone deficiencies experience difficulty sleeping. Progesterone in particular tends to have a very calming influence on the central nervous system, and is a great natural sleep aid. When I put my female patients on progesterone, the quality of their sleep immediately improves.

For men, the hormone testosterone is a great sleep aid. Men who have testosterone deficiencies may develop the Irritable Men Syndrome, which can affect sleep. Likewise, when I put my male patients on testosterone, the quality of their sleep quickly and dramatically improves.

Another leading cause of sleep difficulties is a lack of enough melatonin, a hormone produced by the pineal gland in the brain. Known as the 'hormone of darkness', melatonin is closely associated with our circadian rhythm, the 24-hour biological cycle that governs our sense of day and night, of sleepiness and wakefulness. Evolutionarily, melatonin was released at night after the sun went down, which helped put our ancestors to sleep. When we return to some of the more natural patterns of the earth, we return to caring for our bodies the way we are meant to, which in turn eases and slows the aging process.

Many patients with sleep troubles have a melatonin deficiency. What constitutes a deficiency varies from person to person. As with all hormones, there is a measured deficiency and a functional deficiency, and they are not always the same. Many patients have a true deficiency in terms of being outside of the normal average range; others have a functional deficiency, meaning they need more than the typical average reference. Either condition can impair sleep, and I prescribe melatonin as a supplement to help reduce or remove this obstacle to proper rest.

Of course there are many biochemical reasons why people don't sleep well, and melatonin can't fix them all. We have to get to the core of each patient's problem and work on that issue. It may be tired adrenal glands, it might be stress-released chemicals, it could be diet and nutrition, low thyroid function, a medication the patient takes, or it could be something quite physical, such as pain. It could be obstructive sleep apnea. It could be a combination of things. I work closely with every RVI patient to determine the root cause(s) of their sleep issues and develop a comprehensive, carefully planned response.

THE SLEEP PLAN

The first thing I ask my patients to do is to fill out a history of their sleep habits. I query them about the quality of their sleep. I ask them whether they feel refreshed when they wake in the morning, or whether they sometimes wake up with a headache. I ask them if they feel like they need to nap during the day or if doze off here and there.

Based on this information I give them a sleepiness scale, and if they score high enough I immediately test for obstructive sleep apnea. I must rule this out before we can go any further, because sleep apnea must be treated right away. Until this condition is identified and corrected, afflicted patients will not feel well. They will always be fatigued and unable to lose weight, or even worse, may be putting themselves at risk for a stroke or heart failure.

OBSTRUCTIVE SLEEP APNEA

On the list of physical disorders that affect sleep, the most common is obstructive sleep apnea. This is when people periodically stop breathing because they have an obstruction of the upper airway. Invariably, these patients are heavy snorers. Obstructive sleep apnea is a serious medical condition that predisposes a person to potentially very serious medical problems such as stroke and congestive heart failure.

The obstruction can be caused by a number of factors. Generally the victims have a small lower jaw, a relatively fat tongue, or a collapsing soft pallet. The tongue falls back, or the soft pallet collapses and the airway becomes obstructed. Obstructive sleep apnea can also be made worse by other obstructive issues, such as narrow nasal passages, deviated septums, chronic allergic conditions, edema (swelling) of the mucosal membranes, or adenoids. Any or all of these conditions make it difficult for air to reach the lungs, and could exacerbate the apnea.

Being Overweight

Obesity is one of the main causes of obstructive sleep apnea; indeed, apnea is primarily found in obese men and women. Paradoxically, obesity also is a result of apnea. When you have intermittent or interrupted sleep, it is harder to lose weight. Overeating is also at times a compensation for excessive daytime sleepiness, because we often eat as a way to try and generate energy.

Diagnosing Sleep Apnea

If I suspect that a patient has sleep apnea, I send them to a sleep lab to undergo a sleep study. At the lab the patient is hooked up to an electroencephalograph (to monitor brain waves) and to an electrocardiograph (to monitor heart rate and rhythm). They are also monitored for respiratory rate and the level of oxygen saturation in their blood. This is all recorded along with video of their movements while sleeping.

If there is a diagnosis of obstructive sleep apnea, we have to treat it. One way is to use an air pressure device called a CPAP machine. It's basically a mask hooked up by hose to a small air pump which provides air pressure sufficiently enough to overcome the obstruction. This opens the airway, allowing the patient to breathe normally throughout the night.

Of course, the mask has to be worn nightly - until the sleep apnea is relieved. If the patient loses a lot of weight, they may not need the pump going forward. Some may be able to use a specially fitted mouthpiece called a mandibular advancer that moves the lower jaw and tongue forward. This sometimes creates enough relief of the obstruction to avoid the airway pressure pump.

Surgery is another option. With laser or traditional surgery we can expand the caliber or diameter of the airway by removing some of the soft tissue of the upper pallet. Some people have a very fat uvula, that little tongue in the back of your throat, or just a soft pallet that descends. You can laser off the uvula, or shave down the tissue of the soft palate, and widen the airway.

Surgery may seem like a radical option, but many patients would rather shoot themselves than wear a CPAP breathing device every night. It's not an easy decision, and one you really have to think about carefully. Some people with apnea snore so loudly that their spouse or partner won't sleep in the same room with them. These devices are not attractive, but they greatly improve sleep quality and quantity while making it quiet and possibly improving your relationship with your bed partner. I go through this discussion with many patients, and in the end it comes down to the stubborn fact that you have no choice. Solve the apnea or you aren't going to see the anti-aging results you are hoping for.

The good news is that weight loss can relieve apnea symptoms in about eighty percent of the cases, but patients have to lose enough weight and keep it off, or the apnea will likely return.

The bad news is that there are forms of sleep apnea that aren't related to throat obstructions. One type is called hypopnea, in which breathing is interrupted by dysfunctions in the brain's sleep center. This and other types of apnea are much less common, but they do exist and must be treated.

Regardless of the cause, the end result of sleep apnea is that not enough oxygen goes to the brain, the heart and other vital organs, resulting in tissue damage. Lack of good sleep results in stress, cellular oxidation, and inflammation. This contributes to accelerated aging, and ultimately chronic disease.

LET THERE BE SLEEP

As you can see, there are a slew of things that can lead to sleep issues, from anxiety and hormone levels to diet and insulin levels, all making it tough for people to have a restful night. Once you correct the chemical deficiencies, mitigate the influence of stress and anxiety, balance the hormones, and fix the diet, all of a sudden someone is going to sleep like they've never been able to sleep before, waking up refreshed each morning instead of dragging and fatigued. This solution works because they are returning their body to a more normal, balanced physiology.

The ideal way to sleep is to go to bed, go to sleep, sleep as long as you need to sleep, and then get up without an alarm clock. That's the way our ancestors did it. They didn't have alarm clocks; they worked on circadian rhythms that are natural to the human physiology. Artificially waking ourselves is, well, artificial! It's abnormal. Our body is not made that way, and it's not good for us. Just imagine going to sleep, sleeping restfully through the night unaffected by the ravages of stress and others issues, then waking up, having a nice day, and at the end of it going to sleep again. This should be every person's daily routine.

How many people do you know who live that ideal? Very few, because our society has changed our lifestyle, we've lost respect for our physiology, and we are paying the price. I'm not saying it's realistic to go to bed only when tired and wake only when rested. Most of us need to be somewhere at a certain time each morning; but you know now that you can mindfully manage your sleep; and the results will amaze you.

The upside is that when somebody returns to a reasonably normal sleep pattern, even after a deficit that's been going on for months or years, they bounce back to shape within a week, or even days. It's a quick recovery - providing that's your only issue, of course.

Banked Sleep

Those of us who are very busy and don't get enough sleep during the week will try to "catch up" on vacation or the weekends. But note, you can only bank a limited amount of sleep. The idea is to get adequate sleep every night, or on most nights. If you are sleep deprived, you are probably going to have to get back into a more normal circadian rhythm in order to truly catch up.

29 SECRETS TO A GOOD NIGHT'S SLEEP

If you are having sleep problems, whether you are not able to fall asleep, wake up too often, don't feel well-rested when you wake up in the morning, or simply want to improve the quality and quantity of your sleep, try as many of the following techniques below as possible:

Listen to white noise or relaxation CDs. Some people find the sound of white noise or nature sounds, such as the ocean or forest, to be soothing for sleep. An excellent relaxation/meditation option to listen to before bed is the Insight Audio CD.

Avoid before-bed snacks, particularly grains and sugars. This will raise blood sugar and inhibit sleep. Later, when blood sugar drops too low (hypoglycemia), you might wake up and not be able to fall back asleep.

Sleep in complete darkness or as close as possible. If there is even the tiniest bit of light in the room it can disrupt your circadian rhythm and your pineal gland's production of melatonin and seratonin. There also should be as little light in the bathroom as possible if you get up in the middle of the night. Please whatever you do, keep the light off when you go to the bathroom at night. As soon as you turn on that light you will for that night immediately cease all production of the important sleep aid melatonin.

No TV right before bed. Even better, get the TV out of the bedroom or even out of the house, completely. It is too stimulating to the brain and it will take longer to fall asleep. Also disruptive of pineal gland function for the same reason as above.

Wear socks to bed. Due to the fact that they have the poorest circulation, the feet often feel cold before the rest of the body. A study has shown that this reduces night wakings.

Read something spiritual or religious. This will help to relax. Don't read anything stimulating, such as a mystery or suspense novel, as this may have the opposite effect. In addition, if you are really enjoying a suspenseful book, you might wind up unintentionally reading for hours, instead of going to sleep.

Avoid using loud alarm clocks. It is very stressful on the body to be awoken suddenly. If you are regularly getting enough sleep, they should be unnecessary. I gave up my alarm clock years ago and now use a sun alarm clock, which provides an ideal way to wake up each morning if you can't wake up with the REAL sun. Combining the features of a traditional alarm clock (digital display, AM/FM radio, beeper, snooze button, etc) with a special built-in light that gradually increases in intensity, this amazing clock simulates a natural sunrise. It also includes a sunset feature where the light fades to darkness over time - ideal for anyone who has trouble falling asleep.

Melatonin and its precursors. If behavioral changes do not work, it may be possible to improve sleep by supplementing with the hormone melatonin. However, I would exercise extreme caution in using it, and only as a last resort, as it is a powerful hormone. Ideally it is best to increase levels naturally with exposure to bright sunlight in the daytime (along with full spectrum fluorescent bulbs in the winter) and absolute complete darkness at night. One should get blackout drapes so no light is coming in from the outside. One can also use one of melatonin's precursors, L-tryptophan or 5-hydroxytryptophan (5-HTP). L-tryptophan is the safest and my preference, but must be obtained by prescription only. However, don't be afraid or intimidated by its prescription status. It is just a simple amino acid.

Get to bed as early as possible. Our systems, particularly the adrenals, do a majority of their recharging or recovering during the hours of 11PM and 1AM. In addition, your gallbladder dumps toxins during this same period. If you are awake, the toxins back up into the liver which then secondarily back up into your entire system and cause further disruption of your health. Prior to the widespread use of electricity, people would go to bed shortly after sundown, as most animals do, and which nature intended for humans as well.

Keep the temperature in the bedroom no higher than 70 degrees F. Many people keep their homes and particularly the upstairs bedrooms too hot.

Eat a high-protein snack several hours before bed. This can provide the L-tryptophan need to produce melatonin and serotonin.

Also eat a small piece of fruit. This can help the tryptophan cross the blood-brain barrier.

Reduce or avoid as many drugs as possible. Many medications, both prescription and over-the-counter may have effects on sleep. In most cases, the condition, which caused the drugs to be taken in the first place, can be addressed by following the guidelines elsewhere on this web site.

Avoid caffeine. A recent study showed that in some people, caffeine is not metabolized efficiently and therefore they can feel the effects long after consuming it. So an afternoon cup of coffee (or even tea) will keep some people from falling asleep. Also, some medications, particularly diet pills contain caffeine.

Alarm clocks and other electrical devices. If these devices must be used, keep them as far away from the bed as possible, preferably at least 3 feet.

Avoid alcohol. Although alcohol will make people drowsy, the effect is short lived and people will often wake up several hours later, unable to fall back asleep. Alcohol will also keep you from falling into the deeper stages of sleep, where the body does most of its healing.

Lose weight. Being overweight can increase the risk of sleep apnea, which will prevent a restful nights sleep.

Avoid foods that you may be sensitive to. This is particularly true for dairy and wheat products, as they may have an effect on sleep, such as causing apnea, excess congestion, gastrointestinal upset, and gas, among others.

Don't drink any fluids within 2 hours of going to bed. This will reduce the likelihood of needing to get up and go to the bathroom or at least minimize the frequency.

Take a hot bath, shower or sauna before bed. When body temperature is raised in the late evening, it will fall at bedtime, facilitating sleep.

Remove the clock from view. It will only add to your worry when constantly staring at it... 2 AM...3 AM... 4:30 AM...

Keep Your Bed For Sleeping. If you are used to watching TV or doing work in bed, you may find it harder to relax and to think of the bed as a place to sleep.

Have your adrenals checked by a good natural medicine clinician. Scientists have found that Insomnia may be caused by adrenal stress (Journal of Clinical Endocrinology & Metabolism, August 2001; 86:3787-3794).

If you are menopausal or peri-menopausal, get checked out by a good natural medicine physician. The hormonal changes at this time may cause problems if not properly addressed.

Don't Change Your Bedtime. You should go to bed, and wake up, at the same times each day, even on the weekends. This will help your body to get into a sleep rhythm and make it easier to fall asleep and get up in the morning.

Make certain you are exercising regularly. Exercising for at least 30 minutes everyday can help you fall asleep. However, don't exercise too close to bedtime or it may keep you awake. Studies show exercising in the morning is the best if you can do it.

Journaling. If you often lay in bed with your mind racing, it might be helpful keep a journal and write down your thoughts before bed. Personally, I have been doing this for 15 years, but prefer to do it in the morning when my brain is functioning at its peak and my coritsol levels are high.

Check your bedroom for electro-magnetic fields (EMFs). These can disrupt the pineal gland and the production of melatonin and seratonin, and may have other negative effects as well. To purchase a gauss meter to measure EMFs try Cutcat at 800-497-9516. They have a model for around $40. One doctor even recommends that people pull their circuit breaker before bed to kill all power in the house (Dr. Herbert Ross, author of "Sleep Disorders").

STRESS
MANAGEMENT

CHAPTER 7

Out of control stress is another epidemic in our society, and the havoc it wreaks on our bodies is truly incredible. Stress insidiously manifests itself in many ways; affecting how we feel, look, and function.

http://www.youtube.com/watch?v=zcGKueNP59E

Uncovering how much stress a patient suffers from is a crucial part of the RVI inventory. Dealing with stress is part of the foundation for health and anti-aging. As humans we are not designed to deal with perpetual stress. It's unheard of in terms of our biological history for us to experience stress as something pervasive and relentless. The chronic underlying stress of everyday modern life takes a big toll on the body and its systems.

You'll never be able to eliminate every cause of stress in your life. The trick is to not let it throw obstacles you can't hurdle. You must eliminate what you can, and more importantly, adapt to it and therefore reduce its intensity.

STRESS AGES YOU

First it's important to understand stress; look at where it comes from and how it can damage us, but this is not a simple subject.

http://www.youtube.com/watch?v=aK5HdpUBsao

Some degree of stress is normal and actually necessary. It is, after all, an adaptive mechanism to threatening situations. Without stress you wouldn't react to changes in the environment and dangerous circumstances. This is called acute stress, and it's one of two types, the other being chronic stress.

Acute Stress vs. Chronic Stress

Acute stress is something that we are biologically well equipped to handle. This is the kind of stress we faced in Paleolithic times when we were hunters and gatherers. If a predator tried to attack and eat us, we reacted with the fight or flight response; we would kill the animal or run away. Our bodies flooded with the hormone epinephrine (also known as adrenaline), which increased heart rate, contracted blood vessels, opened air passages, etc. As soon as that moment of threat was over, the system would return to normal.

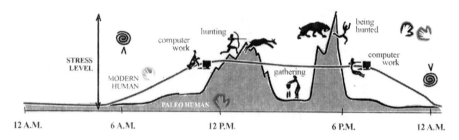

Living The Life: Desk Jockey V. Hunter-Gatherer

What people suffer from in the modern world is chronic stress, which is very different from acute stress. Chronic stress is not a come-and-go event. It is stress you can't seem to get away from; like being

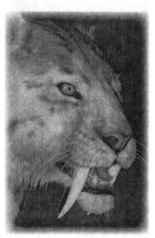

constantly under attack by a predatory animal. In our world it's not a tiger but a tsunami of noise, news, money issues, traffic, and much more - stimulation and anxiety you can't get away from. Maybe it's the threat of a nuclear holocaust, a terrorist attack, a punishing deadline, or an ongoing family crisis - something always eating at you. Never mind what the specific cause might be; it's chronic because it never quits and this has detrimental effects on your mental and physical health.

122

There are two types of coping hormones reflected in our underlying chemistry. Adrenaline is the fight or flight hormone. It gets your heart pumping faster, creates an increase in blood pressure, and gets you ready to run or to fight. It provides the instant surge of energy needed to deal with the crisis at hand.

Cortisol is the other stress coping hormone. It helps when you are under more prolonged stress, affecting things like blood sugar. It provides the energy needed to deal with an extended stress situation - creating a state of constant alert readiness. You are tense and highly aware, but it is not the same heart pumping burst of flight or fight that adrenaline gives. Cortisol helps us deal with non-acute stress, but when non-acute stress remains chronic, it creates a chronic elevation of cortisol in the system. This is unnatural and ultimately damages our physiology.

SOURCES OF STRESS

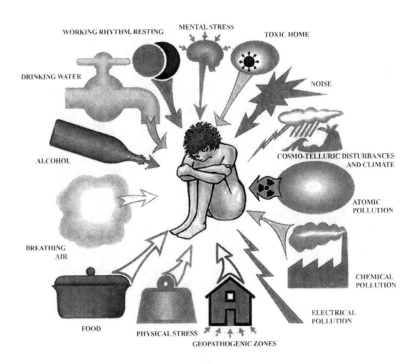

The sources of chronic stress seem to be fairly universal. For most people it boils down to four categories: excessive work, worry over money, dysfunctional relationships, or poor health. Who do you know that doesn't suffer from at least one of these things? Most people do. Some people say - and may think - they don't, but you never know what goes on behind closed doors. Let's just assume these are for the most part universal, and examine them individually.

Work and Money

We live in a society where people work well beyond what their physiology can accommodate. Work typically interferes with all the basics of anti-aging. We don't get the exercise we need because we are seated at our desk for so much of the day. We don't get proper exposure to fresh air and natural light. We work or rush through meals and don't take the time to have social meals. Our world of work is about speed, getting it done fast and getting on with it. That is disruptive to our physiology.

Money is a closely related generator of stress, driving us to work longer hours. It comes with a large helping of emotional issues like anxiety and fear. Today there are many people who work two jobs and families in which both adults must work just to have a lifestyle that only a generation ago was provided by one job per household. There are also additional family stresses. Women who enter the work force have less time and energy for family, children, and themselves.

The stressors of work can add up. You face traffic and pollution making your way to and from work each day. By the time you get home, you can't stop thinking about the boss or client who is acting like a jerk; you may be aggravated or worried and do not sleep well. Perhaps you're working late and stay busy until twenty minutes before you go to bed, leaving you unable to fall asleep. The stress of work itself, with its demands of energy and hours, added to anxiety about how you'll pay for everything on your and your family's need and wish lists, not to mention what the future economy might bring, is enough to keep anyone awake on any given night. Remember, these sources of stress are universal. It's important and helpful to keep in mind that you are not alone. We all face these demands and stresses every day. It's what you do to prepare for, manage, cope with, and balance stress that will help you sleep better, function more efficiently, and feel better while doing it.

Are You a 'Type A'?

Even if you're successful at work and money is not a big concern, that doesn't mean you are immune to stress. Frequently, the opposite is true. You've heard of the 'Type A' personality? The Type A personality is all go, go, go, work, work, work, and stress, stress, stress. These people experience a roller coaster of

http://www.youtube.
com/watch?v=dY79
mq5pxpA

stress, up and down, with adrenaline levels on high the majority of the time. It's like facing a predator around every bend, down every corridor, and at the other end of every phone call.

The Type A personality releases high levels of catecholamines - adrenaline and norepinephrine. This is dangerous because these constrict blood vessels so much that blood is redirected to the essential organs for flight or fight - the heart, the brain, and the muscles. This causes chronic vasoconstriction, which means increased heart rate and increased blood pressure. When that becomes continuous over time it creates secondary problems, such as cardiovascular disease.

The advent of the 24-hour day makes all of this even worse. We now have around-the-clock noise, music, information, cell phones, texting, and portable entertainment devices. This endless stimulation is a huge contributor to stress, right down to its impact on work and sleep.

Relationships

After work and money comes relationships, which are always a big source of stress. Even when the friendships, love and family ties in your life are healthy, relationships mean responsibility, obligation, and concern. Relationships of any kind (mother, father, husband, wife, boyfriend, girlfriend, brother, sister, friend, etc.) mean endless complications of compromise and co-existence. This is another wrinkle in stress, moving it from the physical to the emotional, just as the physical effects of being over-worked transform into the emotional effects of worrying about money.

Bottled-up, unresolved, chronic, emotional conflict leads to harmful stress. The same goes for guilt, anger, and fear, emotions typically involved in unresolved relationship issues. These are all emotions that create tremendous, pervasive stress. If you know anyone who is living in or struggling to get out of a bad relationship, chances are they are juggling these powerful emotions and you can observe that they are always stressed.

Then there is love. Whatever love is, one of the most useful things it does is to help mitigate stress. Individuals who have strong ties to family and friends tend to live longer than loners. Even argumentative families and complicated relationships, as long as they have a mechanism for conflict resolution, offer health benefits.

Health

Finally, there is stress related to health. Poor health in and of itself is a cause of stress. This creates a downward, self-fulfilling spiral, since ongoing stress has a negative effect on overall health. Many people are stressed out because they don't feel well, and a lot of people don't feel well because they are stressed.

Health in this sense is closely related to depression and self-esteem, especially when it comes to our sense of energy and how we appear. If you feel lackluster and have low energy due to poor health, you feel depressed. If you believe you also look unattractive, even more stress occurs.

Conversely, when you feel better about yourself, you're less stressed out. Unfortunately, those who have low self-esteem find it very hard to feel good about themselves. If this sense of weak self-worth leads to feeling that life has no meaning or purpose, the result is extreme stress and accelerated aging. It is essential to break this cycle, or it just keeps going.

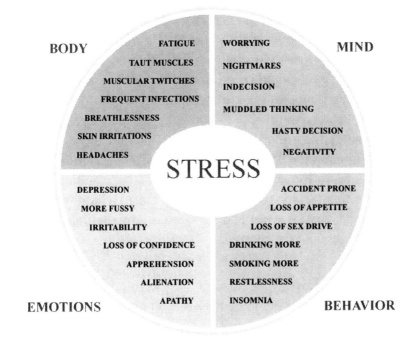

Stress symptoms

HOW WE DETERMINE STRESS LEVELS

In light of the complexity of stress, I work with my patients at RVI on a number of different levels. First and foremost I try to measure how much their exposure to prolonged stress has affected their ability to manage short-term stress. To begin, we measure where patients are in terms of adrenal function; a key indicator of stress. I then take a patient history. This is a detailed inventory of their stress and stress factors, how these factors affect their life, and what their personal, unique sources of stress are.

http://www.youtube.com/watch?v=r2x WaiSHUk8

Checking the Adrenals

The adrenal stress index, which is how we describe the functioning of the adrenal gland in response to stress, is a highly revelatory test for examining how stress physically affects a patient. The way humans deal with stress, biologically, is primarily through the adrenal glands. These glands sit on top of the kidneys and release hormones such as cortisol and catecholamines (e.g. epinephrine, aka adrenaline, and norepinephrine) that fire up the body for action in response to stress. If you are constantly under stress, your adrenal glands become exhausted and no longer respond normally. The resulting adrenal fatigue leads to a plethora of negative symptoms, including tiredness, poor sleep, cravings for sweet and salty foods, low stamina, difficulty concentrating, and so forth.

While the adrenal stress index itself is important, the ultimate test is how the patient feels. If my patient says, "Oh man, I'm stressed out," and I take their history and see signs and symptoms of suffering, this is more a confirmation of maladaptive stress than any adrenal test. If a patient suffering the symptoms of adrenal exhaustion actually has an impaired adrenal stress index, then I prescribe a specific program

ADRENAL EXHAUSTION SURVEY SAMPLE

Instructions:
Rate the occurrence of each symptom according to the scale. and then calculate your total score below.

RATING SCALE

0 - Never	1 - Seldom		2 - Occasionally
3 - Frequently	4 - Infrequently but with Severe Symptoms		5 - Almost Always

Fatigue	Craving for sweets
Exhaustion	Less than normal perspiration
Nervousness, irritability, anxiety	Food and other allergies
Depression	Low blood pressure
Inability to concentrate	Lightheadedness on standing up
Poor Memory	Difficulty overcoming infections
Headaches	Severe or recurrent stresses
Always feel cold (abnormally low body temperature)	Hypoglycemia (especially if resistant to normal measures. require persistent attention)
Premenstrual symptoms (especially if resistant to normal measures or requiring persistent attention)	Slow recovery from any kind of stress (exercise. overwork. mental strain, inadequate sleep, emotional trauma, injury, surgery)

TOTAL SCORE:

INTERPRETING YOUR SCORES:

If you score is in the range of 1-10, this may indicate a mild imbalance.

If you score is in the range of 11-20, this may indicate a moderate imbalance.

If you score is in the range of 21-34, this may indicate a severe imbalance.

If you score is over 35, this may indicate a critical imbalance.

nourishing the adrenals and restoring adrenal adaptation. I also balance each patient's cortisol level by either providing support for their cortisol if it's too low, or by lowering it if it's too high.

SAMPLE LIFESTYLE THERAPY OPTIONS

Lifestyle therapy options:
Stress / Adrenal - Rx and Edu

STRESS AND ADRENAL

Stress / Adrenal Details Glycemic control through diet,
High / Low Cortisol States. Low States, Lifestyle and
Environmental Recommendations and Mental/Emotional / Spiritual

LOW CORTISOL STATES	DOSAGE
Hydrocortisone	7am-8am - 12.5mg, 11am-12noon - 5mg, 3pm-4pm - 2.5mg

GLYCEMIC CONTROL

- Whole foods
- Carbohydrate / protein balance
- Glycemic load 10 or less
- Adequate protein as instructed
- No sugar
- No caffeine

HIGH OR LOW CORTISOL STATES	DOSAGE
Glucobalance	Qty 1. 3 times daily with meals
Extra Vitamin B - 5 (Pantothenic acid)	500mg 2 times daily with meals
Adreset	Qty 1, 2 times daily, last one before 3 pm

LIFESTYLE AND ENVIRONMENTAL RECOMMENDATIONS

	Discussed with patient!
Adequate but not excessive exercise	Yes
Adequate Sleep	Yes
Art / music / nature: things and places of beauty	Yes
Breath clean air and drink clean water	Yes
Get outdoors and have some full spectrum lighting	Yes
Home improvements: making your place a sanctuary	Yes
Recreation / fun	Yes
Relaxation exercise / meditation / breathing	Yes

MENTAL / EMOTIONAL / SPIRITUAL RECOMMENDATIONS

Nurturing / affection / love	Discussed with patient!
Fun / laughter	Yes
Cultivating community and relationships: people, pets, plants	Yes

Resolving chronic emotional conflicts best you can: anger, fear, depression, guilt consider therapy to work out conflicts	Yes
Build self esteem	Yes
The hardy personality	Yes
Find meaning / purpose	Yes
MORE INFO	

Prescriptions Given
- GlucoBalance Capsule Capsule - 90 Capsule (0 refills)
- Vitamin B5 500 Milligram Capsule - 0 Capsule (0 refills)

THE REJUVALIFE VITALITY INSTITUTE (RVI) PROGRAM: LEARNING TO DEAL WITH IT

It is absolutely essential to find a way to realistically deal with the stresses in life. Doing so comes down to a series of conscious decisions on your part. First, become aware of your own sources of stress, and then modify your behavior to mitigate their effects. This is especially important for RVI patients as they embark on the journey they have come to me for help with.

Countless books have been written about how to deal with stress, how to relax, find inner peace, and so forth. By and large these books approach stress from two points of view: changing your environment to reduce stress, or changing your reaction to stress to make it less harmful. The sage advice of these books comes down to two things: change your life or change your attitude.

Changing Lifestyle

It's nearly impossible to avoid or even mitigate every situation that produces stress in our lives. The thing to do is sit down and take an inventory, just as I do with my RVI patients, and then do what you can to alter the worst sources of stress for the better.

Some things you can do (or not do) are obvious. Stop rushing through meals. It's not just about what you eat, but how you eat. We need to relish the ritual of dining, of nourishing our bodies and minds at the same time. Dining should be a process whereby you prepare for the meal by relaxing yourself. Relaxation improves digestion, which improves your ability to enjoy and benefit from your food.

I also recommend making eating an opportunity for social connectivity rather than solitary confinement. Eating is designed to be a social event. Our ancestors didn't just catch their food and sit and eat it. Hunters and gatherers would collectively go out and get the food, then bring it back to wherever they were encamped, where the community would collectively clean and prepare it for their group dining experience. This may seem like a small, unimportant thing in today's hectic world, especially in light of the serious challenges that many people face; but that is exactly my point. To survive the crush of our modern world, we must mitigate the thousand pinpricks of stress that collectively wear us down - one small stressor at a time. They add up, and you'd be surprised how much good even a little stress reduction can do.

Take light, for example. Today's workday is disruptive to many simple things, and getting enough natural light is one of them. People are cooped up in offices with artificial lighting all day. They rarely get outside for exposure to full-spectrum lighting. Just step outside, take a walk, go to the park, walk around the block a couple of times; try to get outdoors for thirty minutes each day. Spending too much time under artificial light is stressful.

Exercise is one of the most effective stress relievers available. It reduces stress and improves conditions in every system of the body. Some exercise every day is essential to reducing our overall level of stress. Yoga and other Eastern forms of exercise are especially conducive to relaxation, with their attention to mental relaxation (meditation) and deep breathing. The best exercises, of course, are the ones you most enjoy doing.

Other major lifestyle issues, such as relationships and career, call for dealing with each stress at the source. End a relationship that is killing you or find a job that makes you feel happy, inspired and fulfilled. These are not things you can do overnight, but they are possible. Empower yourself. The all-important first step is making a conscious decision to change.

Realistically, major life shifts are often easier said than done, and many people face situations that are difficult to change. This is where the inner game comes into play. In the end, much of how stressful situations affect our health is determined by how we react to them. Bottom line, attitude is critical.

A great many studies show that people who have positive attitudes - those who are highly optimistic (or happily married, or who have large groups of relatives and friends to interact with, have a loving pet, or who find their work satisfying and fulfilling) tend to live longer, heal faster, get sick less often, and so forth. They are less debilitated by the stress that we all face. The opposite is a negative mindset, specifically one overwhelmed by fear. Once the adrenals start to kick in, and cortisol and catecholamines start to rise, there are emotional consequences - mostly fear. People are scared when they are stressed, and stressed when they are scared.

All of this leads us to the ultimate stress release, which is happiness. We will discuss this idea in greater detail later, but for now, it's an important concept to keep in mind. When it comes to stress relief, recreation and fun are extremely important. With most of my patients, I look at them and say, "So, what do you do for fun?" A lot of them need to seriously think for several beats before they can pin down what they do for fun. This is sad yet common.

What I have learned (and seen, time and again), is that a happy life is a balanced life in which you do something for yourself every day. It's not a magical solution, but it will help. If it makes you happy, your body chemistry will reflect it by producing less cortisol and epinephrine. The creation or appreciation of art, music, nature, things and places of beauty are experiences that help people enjoy life and mitigate stress.

The Home Sanctuary

If you think I am suggesting that happiness can be a sanctuary from the stress of daily life, you are correct. With my patients at RVI I take this to its literal conclusion, and what I suggest to all of them is to make home improvements. Make your home a sanctuary.

A very common problem is that many people have no oasis of calm, and if you live in a chaotic environment it's hard to relax. If you have a highly demanding job, you may not want to come home and put things away. The result is a messy home, which creates more stress. Think about it. Unless you are totally oblivious to everything around you, you become part of the chaos.

You can test this very easily. Go to a nice, tranquil environment, with soft sounds, beautiful things, and pleasing smells. Spend ten minutes there and think about how you feel. Then walk into an office that is a total mess, with papers strewn all over the place, or into a bedroom with underwear and socks and dirty dishes on the floor, and see how you feel. You won't have to go any further. The point here is that your home is only a sanctuary if it's conducive, in a ritual way, to peaceful, calming relaxation. It's pretty simple. If you want to feel better, spend time in an environment conducive to feeling better. If you've got clutter, clean it up; make yourself a place to go where you know you can relax. You'd be shocked to know that most people don't have such a place. I encourage RVI patients to create that oasis as another way to mitigate stress.

Stress reduction in your home and in general will help you sleep better, feel better because you're truly rested, function better because you aren't tired all the time, and as a result, experience less stress because you're on top of things. When you are calm and on top of things you are happy, which also helps to keep stress at bay.

The cycle is clear, but not always easy to accomplish, which is why at RVI we begin with the detailed inventories for each patient and then design each recovery and anti-aging program specific to individual needs.

Avoid Drugs

One thing I don't encourage is the use of drugs (either prescription or illegal) as a coping mechanism. This should seem obvious, but when people are looking for relief, common sense often flies out the window. When you're feeling the ravages of stress, it's easy to think that chemical relief is appropriate. After all, the stress has to be worse than the medication, right? Wrong. Outside the medically proven benefits of a small amount of alcohol, I see no benefits to taking drugs to deal with stress - and this runs the gamut from marijuana to Xanax. In the short term they can certainly relieve symptoms of stress. They can get someone really relaxed, and they can modulate pain. While this is all true, they are not beneficial to your health vis-à-vis long-term stress. Drugs solve nothing long-term and typically have negative, if not dangerous, side effects, including addictions that create their own set of stressful problems.

You must alter the cause of stress, and if you can't change the cause, you can learn to mitigate its effects naturally; through exercise, meditation, socializing, creating a personal sanctuary, etc. If you can't mitigate stress through introspection and self-help, then you may need to seek outside counseling in the form of a psychologist or therapist. Cognitive behavioral therapy is very effective for many people.

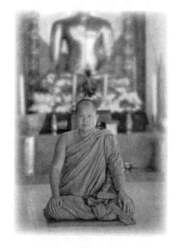

The important thing to realize is that stress is destructive, and that no anti-aging program will work if you have chronic, pervasive stress. Stress kills - slowly but surely. It wreaks havoc through our hormones, and basically all of our biological systems.

The scary fact is that this chronic, pervasive stress is rampant in our society and very hard to escape. It seems to be the rule, rather than the exception. What we are trying to do in anti-aging is to make it the exception rather than the rule. By altering our environment and behavior we create a more balanced life conducive to slow, healthy aging.

CHANGING HABITS: WHAT IT TAKES TO SUCCEED

CHAPTER 8

As mentioned earlier, much of what we are trying to address in anti-aging is induced by years of poor lifestyle choices and basic bad habits. For many people, their unhealthy situation isn't entirely their fault, because they are only doing what they've been taught. There are plenty of people, however, who know better and yet repeat bad behavior, because habits are hard to break and new, good habits are difficult to establish.

Eating habits are the first behaviors we want to change, and we have to start making changes immediately for any anti-aging program to work. If my patients have hormone issues, I treat these issues simultaneously. Once we have the test results, hormone treatment is simple; a matter of taking pills, rubbing on gels or creams, or self-administering painless injections. I prefer to start my patients on the right lifestyle path from day one, so the anti-aging process is not delayed or undermined.

http://www.youtube.com/watch?v=BwZA2xuxYTA

The path to wellness and successful age management must include the entire foundation - of diet, exercise, sleep, and stress management. Without changing bad habits, patients inevitably get discouraged, because other therapies will not meet their expectations, and any improvement is short-lived.

Of course, patients aren't expected to do everything in every category right away. We work gradually, based on what I estimate they can do initially, and add incrementally, so with my guidance they stay on track with best odds of being successful. Determining the best balance and timing for each patient is a challenge. If people try to do too much too soon, they often have to take steps back, and re-adjust.

TREATMENT GOALS	
DECREASE PERCENT BODY FAT	INCREASE LEAN BODY MASS
IMPROVE MUSCLE STRENGTH	IMPROVE POST EXERCISE RECOVERY
INCREASE LIBIDO	IMPROVE QUALITY OF SKIN
IMPROVE UPON ERECTIONS	DECREASE FREQUENCY OF COLDS
IMPROVE ON HAIR CONDITION	INCREASE PHYSICAL ENERGY
IMPROVE MEMORY	INCREASE MENTAL ENERGY
INCREASE MENTAL ALERTNESS	IMPROVE UPON SLEEP
IMPROVE UPON MOOD	IMPROVE ON MILD DEPRESSION
	DECREASE MENOPAUSE SYMPTOMS

MANAGING EXPECTATIONS

Success with anti-aging has a lot to do with realistic expectations. Nothing is more disheartening than failing to meet goals. Some people believe treatment will re-grow all their hair, save their marriage, or help them make another million dollars in the coming year - in these cases I have to tell them what they can reasonably expect to achieve. You'd be surprised how many people have unrealistic expectations. They want instant, dramatic improvement, and that just doesn't happen. Changing a lifetime of bad habits and transforming them into good ones is like turning a giant ocean liner. You can't turn it on a dime, but once you make the turn, the momentum is in your favor.

Education is key to managing expectations. Many doctors don't take the time to fully discuss things with their patients. This is unfortunate, because people often form habits based on incorrect information and if a doctor doesn't take the time to help them form new ones, not much will change. Traditional medical practitioners often just give patients a few pills (prescription medication) and wish them good luck. They use pharmacology to treat patients without addressing the underlying, functional imbalances.

I believe it is paramount to get patients off all but the most vital medications. I take the time to instruct, re-train, and educate them about how to achieve their goals. Good health doesn't come in a pill, and everyone is different. Some patients change quickly while others take a long time to wean off their medications. Regardless of the method, patients must really change their fundamental behaviors if they want to succeed with anti-aging treatments.

AM EVALUATION PHASE VISIT

Age Management Subjective

AGE MANAGEMENT EVALUATION PHASE PRE-VISIT CHECK LIST	ANSWER
Questionnaires all completed, signed, dated, and scanned into Nextech	Yes
Forms all completed, signed, dated, and witnessed and scanned into Nextech	Yes
Nexweb forms all completed in EMR prior to visit	Yes
Lab results received and reviewed by MD	Yes
Patient Questionnaires received and reviewed by MD	Yes

Age Management Interview/Review Patient documents reviewed and detailed interview conducted by MD.

Age Management Objective

LAB COLLECTION (QUEST)				REVIEWED
• Comprehensive Panel				Yes
LAB COLLECTION (REFERENCE LABS)				**REVIEWED**
• ASI				Yes
• Urine GH				Yes
VITALS AM				
• Height	6'0"	• Heart Rate	85	• Waist Circumference	38
• Weight	220	• Temp	98.5	• Hip Circumference	34
• Blood Pressure	140/95	• BMI	28	• Waist to Hip Ratio	1.12

Age Management Assessment

AGE MANAGEMENT ASSESSMENT: LIFESTYLE ISSUES			
• Diet and Nutrition	Yes	• Sleep	Yes
• Exercise	Yes	• Strevss	Yes

AGE MANAGEMENT ASSESSMENT: OTHER PROBLEMS

• Adrenal Maladaptation / Fatigue	Yes	• High risk category for chronic disease (heart, cancer, diabetes, Alzheimer's, etc)	Yes
• Chronic Stress	Yes		
• Sleep disorder	Yes	• Family history of Alzheimer's disease	Yes
• Sleep Deprivation / inadequate sleep	Yes		
		• BPH without obstruction	Yes
• Obstructive sleep apnea	Yes	• Hypertension	Yes
• Gut dysbiosis	Yes	• Increased CRP	Yes
• Hormone Deficiencies	Yes	• Increased Homocystine	Yes
• Hormone Imbalance	Yes	• Insulin resistant	Yes
• Testosterone (androgen) deficiency	Yes	• Osteo-Arthritis	Yes
		• Obesity	Yes
• Adult growth hormone deficiency		• Truncal / Visceral obesity	Yes
		• Reduced Exercise capacity	Yes
• Hypothyroidism (clinical or subclinical)		• Adverse cardiac risk profile	Yes
		• Decreased energy and vitality	Yes
• Metabolic Syndrome (syndrome x)			
• Hyperinsulinemia (obesity related)			

AGE MANAGEMENT EVALUATION HORMONE IMBALANCES/DEFICINCIES

• Cortisol	Yes	• Estradiol	Yes	• Melatonin	Yes	• Testosterone	Yes
• DHEA	Yes	• HGH	Yes	• Pregnenolone	Yes	• Thyroid	Yes

Age Management Diagnosis Codes

• Abnormal Fasting glucose - 790.21	• Hypercholesterolemia - 272.1
• Adrenal Insufficiency - 255.4	• Hyperlipidemia - 272
• Adult Growth Hormone Deficiency - 253.3	• Hypogonadism - 257.2
	• Hypothyroidism - 242.9
• Adverse Cardiac Risk Profile	• Increased CRP - 790.95
• Decreased Energy and Vitality	• Insomnia - 780.52
• Decreased Libido - 302.71	• Insulin Resistance - 277.7
• Decreased Muscular Strength	• Obesity - 278.02
• Dyslipidemia - 272	• Obstructive Sleep Apnea - 780.53
• Family History CAD - v17.4	• Reduced Exercise Capacity
• Family History Cancer - v16.9	• Screening for Diabetes -v77.1
• Family History Diabetes - v18.0	• Screening for lipid disorders - v77.91

• Family History Osteoporosis - v17.81	• Screening for thyroid disorders - v77.0
• Family Hx of Alzheimer's Disease	• Screening for unspecified
• Fatigue - 780.79	condition - v82.9
• Hormone Imbalance - 259.9	• Sleep disturbance - 780.5

More Info

- 790.2 - Abnormal Fasting Glucose
- 255.4 - Adrenal Insufficiency/CORTICOADRENAL INSUFFIC
- 253.3 - Adult Growth Hormone Def/PITUITARY DWARFISM
- 302.71 - Decreased Libido/HYPOACTIVE SEXUAL DESIRE
- 272 - Hyperlipidemia
- V17.4 - Family HX Cardiovas Dis OT
- V18.0 - Family HX Diabetes Mellitus
- V16.9 - Family History Cancer
- V17.81 - Family HX Osteoper
- 780.79 - Fatigue
- 259.9 - Hormone Inbalance/ENDOCRINE DISORDER UNSPEC
- 272.1 - Hypercholesterolemia
- 257.2 - Hypoandrogenism/TESTICULAR HYPOFUNCTN OT
- 242.9 - Hyperthyroidism
- 790.95 - Elevated CRP
- 780.5 - Insomnia/Sleep Disturbances
- 277.7 - Insulin Resistance/DYSMETABOLIC SYNDROME X
- 278.02 - Overweight
- 780.53 - Obstructive Sleep Apnea/HYPERSOMNIA W SLEEP APN UNS
- V77.1 - Screening for Diabetes Mellitus
- V77.91 - Screening for Lipoid Disorder
- V77.0 - Screening for Thyroid Disorder
- V82.9 - Screening for Condition Unspec

Age Management Evaluation Phase Recommended Treatment Plan

• Hormone Replacement Therapy	• Sleep
• Adrenal Fatigue	• Insulin Resistance
• Nutrition	• Weight Management
• Supplementation	• Screening Tests
• Exercise	• Reference lab testing

Evaluation Phase Recommended Hormone Replacement Therapy		
• Testosterone	• HGH	• DHEA
• Thyroid	• HCG	
• Pregnenolone	• Anastrazole	
Nutrition Plan		
• Diet Prescription	• Nutritionist Consultation	
Recommended Diagnostic Screenings		
• Rapid CT Scan of Heart for Calcium Score		
Adrenal Fatigue		
• Adrenal Treatment Plan	• Stress Reduction	
Supplementation Plan		
• Supplement List		
Insulin Resistance Plan		
• Lifestyle improvement	• Hormone Replacement Therapy	• Medication
Sleep Plan		
• Sleep Education	• Sleep Aids	• Sleep Study
Weight Management Plan		
• Weight Mgmt Program		
Recommended Reference Lab Tests		
• ASI	• Alcat comp 1	• NutraEval
The patient will sign up for treatment phase today.	Yes	

How We Begin

Once a patient decides to work with me, and we've gone through all the inventories and testing described above, I give them a list of what they need to work on, a basic anti-aging blueprint. They may be stronger in certain categories than others, but what they need to do every day is go through their list and work on everything they can. Over time they gradually accomplish more and more. This builds up a sense of self-confidence and self-esteem that carries them through the later changes and challenges that are more difficult to master.

To be successful, patients must develop what I call a 'hearty personality'. If you have a hearty personality it means you are someone who is ready to face the challenges of everyday life along with the changes required for an anti-aging program.

Most of us, with very few exceptions, are faced with many challenges each day; these are not going to go away. I tell my patients that they must develop the ability to meet challenges, and there are strategies they can learn to make those challenges easier to manage.

The first thing you must do to be successful in achieving any goal - and develop a hearty personality - is to make a commitment to achieve that goal. If you don't commit to accomplishing your goals, you won't. It's that simple.

This is different from having a solid plan. You need that as well. Many people verbalize their desires and even map out their program plan, but lack the commitment to see it through. You must commit to all the steps to truly implement and carry out the plan.

Another concept people need to understand as they move through an anti-aging program, is that there are going to be more obstacles than expected. A patient may be doing very well on the program, with everything going their way, when suddenly out of the blue they are involved in a freak car accident. Suddenly, they're in the hospital focused on recovery from injuries and unable to exercise. Everything is thrown off. If they don't have a hearty personality, this can do some people in.

Make no mistake, obstacles will come. You've got to have an attitude that lets you start over every day. Each morning is a new opportunity to be better, no matter what happened to you yesterday. If you had three glasses of wine and a double cheeseburger yesterday, then today you must get back on track. You need to have a hearty personality to do that.

The Hearty Personality

What exactly is a hearty personality? It means being thick-skinned, at least to a certain degree. In our society today, the assaults on our psyche are so relentless that it's difficult to deal with them without being strong. This doesn't mean you should live your life as a limp noodle, not caring about what's happening, or stiff as a ramrod, where you don't feel anything or offer any flexibility. There has to be balance.

Much of a hearty personality is about self-confidence. Those who take everything personally, generally have low self-confidence and low self-esteem. It's hard for these people to do well on the kinds of anti-aging programs I prescribe, but when I can help these people develop a heartier personality, they can get through the obstacles in their own paths and keep going.

THE BENEFITS OF SLOW AND STEADY

The best approach to all of this is taking things one step at a time. By moving forward at a gradual pace, with changes that can be realistically achieved, patients start to feel better about themselves mentally and physically, thus becoming more resilient. This early success begets further success.

It's a bit of a paradox. You want to make yourself aware of and sensitive to the voice within when it comes to things like good food, exercise, sleep, and coping with stress. At the same time, however, you have to desensitize yourself to some of the interferences that may hamper your ability to remain focused and committed. It isn't easy, but this will greatly benefit you over time.

Part of the ability to sustain yourself through challenges comes from changing yourself in a gradual, incremental way. You'll probably never get rid of all your stress sources, but if you start adding good behaviors on a daily basis, it will help you handle a lot of the tough stuff much better.

That Elusive Thing Called Purpose

You need nothing short of a full commitment to achieve your goals. You're going to have to figure out the big goal behind your smaller goals and their achievement. It means finding meaning and purpose. This is a very deep, philosophical concept, but it's also very important.

Personally, I don't know anybody who can do well with anti-aging - or anything else that requires commitment - without meaning and purpose. Human beings are driven by meaning and purpose, and the lack of it makes it very hard to achieve anything. You end up floundering through life. With meaning and purpose you have direction and goals, and can take charge of your life. If you don't have it, then any road will do and you could end up anywhere, or nowhere. Decide where you want to go.

Decide Where You Want To Go

I tell my patients to think about their meaning and purpose in life. If they discover it, they feel better about themselves. If they haven't discovered it yet, they really need to work on it. Sometimes it's a life-long process. Sometimes just the act of trying to figure it all out is helpful. People learn more about themselves, their strengths and weaknesses - and improve themselves in general. The process itself is very valuable.

Find the driven personality within yourself. We can call it the "artistic personality." Artists have a burning ambition to produce a certain kind of art, a vision they stick to regardless of family relationships, personal finances, or any other stress. They remain focused. Contrast this with someone that has no particular drive or goal such as the lackadaisical, bemused type who find things interesting or fun but hasn't set any objectives. It's very hard for this type to impose new changes or modify their habits to achieve anything.

People who set goals for themselves are more likely to produce the behaviors necessary to achieve those goals. People with meaning and purpose understand this, and have the hearty personality needed to persevere. The person without a goal won't care enough when challenges arrive. Their internal voice might say something like, "What's the difference? Maybe I'll die a little younger, maybe I'll get sick, but who cares? I'll go and have that beer now, and let the future take care of itself." His or her pattern of behavior is not programmed to succeed because it's not goal driven.

Bad Habits or Addictions?

To some degree, all habits have addictive components to them, both physiological and psychological. It's much harder to break a habit when there is a very strong physiological component, because then you've got to deal with the chemistry of addiction. Certain kinds of food addictions are powerful for the same reason. There is a true physiological dependence on a chemical substance.

Addictions that are purely psychological can be powerful as well, but rarely are they as potent as when there is a strong physiologic element present. Have you heard of people getting addicted to exercise? Well they do, and partly because both psychological and physiological elements are involved. When you exercise you really like the way you feel about yourself, which reinforces the behavior. You simultaneously have a physiological response. During exercise you release a variety of chemicals such as endorphins, which make you feel better. Levels of neurotransmitters such as serotonin and dopamine also tend to improve. Biochemical changes from exercise also mitigate stress. All these chemical reactions foster an addiction - in this case a good one - that is helped along by that rush of feeling better from exercise.

The same mix of psychological components and body chemistry is true of eating, as well. The dining experience is a psychological and subjective pleasure, but you can become physically addicted to many substances in food, including salt, fat, and sugar, because they change your brain and body chemistry.

To a very real extent, the relationship between habit and addiction can be seen as a matter of degree, along the same continuum. While this may be an over-simplification, habits can clearly be viewed as psychological addictions with a basis in physiology.

All behaviors affect body chemistry and vice versa. When you form a new habit, it creates new neural pathways. These biochemical patterns are associated with being comfortable with that activity. In order to become comfortable with an alternative activity, your brain must carve different neural pathways in order to become equally comfortable with the new behavior.

You might ask, "So are all habits actually addictions?" In terms of basic neurophysiology, you could say they potentially are. Every habit you form, in some microscopic way, changes your basic brain chemistry, and therefore is potentially an addiction; but in practical terms, the changing of everyday habits is not the same as breaking an addiction, not in the usual sense of that word. People with addictions face unstoppable cravings that they can't control or change easily. This is why there is an entire industry based on helping people free themselves from chemical addictions. Chemical addiction is why it's harder to quit consuming sugar than it is to go to the gym for half an hour.

Nonetheless, you are going to have to break certain habits and replace them with better ones. If your vice is sugar, then you'll need to use better nutrition as a replacement and with better nutrition you'll create a healthier insulin response curve. When you change your eating habits, the roller coaster stabilizes. This is what happens when you begin to chip away at bad habits.

THE OPTIMIST CLUB

Another way to look at this is within the emotional paradigm of optimism. Individuals who are optimistic do better with change. People who are pessimistic usually have some element of depression at play. They have a depressed mood, so they are not going to be as receptive to new ideas and behaviors.

Generally speaking, positive attitudes are healthier than negative ones, and pessimistic people tend to age more rapidly. This is only logical. If you are negative by nature, what is that going to affect? First, it's going to affect your brain chemistry by dampening your neural activity, which happens with any element of depression. Negative people tend toward rejection of new things, so they're less open to potentially beneficial changes. Second, people who are depressed are going to have problems with social interaction, connectivity, and relationships, and those problems all lead to more stress.

In order to succeed with an anti-aging program, you need a sense of purpose and meaning, and the positive energy that goes with it. You need a hearty personality, which means one that is neither weak nor rigid, but one that can move forward in a cycle of gradual improvement, growing self-confidence, and meaningful purpose. Find these strengths within yourself and you are halfway home. In the end, it leads to that ultimate goal which is as simple as it is elusive: happiness.

Try This!
Here's a simple exercise to demonstrate the power of habit: Sit up straight in your chair and cross your hands in your lap. Remain sitting until you feel fairly comfortable. Now, change your hands by crossing them the other way. Does this feel comfortable? Probably not.

When you crossed your hands the first time you spontaneously placed them that way because it was the most comfortable position based on a habit you've formed over time. If you do it another way, you feel even less comfortable.

If you want to feel just as comfortable with your hands crossed the second way, you'll have to change the habit. Practically speaking, that means you'll have to do it the new way every time you cross your arms for about three weeks - every day, several times a day. At that point the new way will feel about as comfortable as the old way. New neural pathways will have established themselves in your brain, creating the chemical signature of a new habit.

This is a simple way to show how even a simple habit is not easy to change. How long does it take to make major behavioral changes? As long as it takes for you to feel comfortable with each new habit - each person is different. Some people can make major changes in three weeks, some people take three months, and some people take a year, but no one can change if they give up.

On the other hand, you have nothing to fear but change. We are not talking about learning something really new, like how to play the piano, but about changing relatively simple behaviors that are easy to perform. There's not a lot of difference between the ability to eat organic food rather than eat processed foods. Your ability or capacity to perform the task is not the problem. Making the change is the problem; it's hard, but essential.

Age management medicine is as much about learning to change behaviors as it is about any particular treatment prescribed. Changing personal behavior is a key component to anti-aging, because a patient who doesn't change falls back into the same unhealthy patterns that led them to seek anti-aging treatments in the first place.

Doctors who do this kind of work must be very patient and help people understand the need for change, while at the same time help patients build realistic expectations. Change has to take place gradually in each area of our foundation: diet, exercise. sleep, and stress management.

Anti-aging success comes from being a partner in the process. I can advise and instruct patients on what to do, how to do it, and why they need to do it, but they have to make the changes themselves. I have this conversation with every patient, so they understand that if they don't make any changes, they just won't get there. There are many people who unfortunately won't change enough to reach all of their expectations. My obligation is to put the cards on the table, and show you that what you reap truly depends on what you sow.

HORMONE THERAPY

CHAPTER 9

One of the clearest markers of aging is declining hormone levels. Whereas hormones are plentiful when we are young and vital, their levels recede as we grow older, especially after the age of forty. Restoring hormones to more youthful levels is an essential and powerful component of anti-aging medicine.

The vitality that hormone replacement brings back to the average person is, in most cases, extraordinary. It restores all the attributes of youth that vanish in tandem with disappearing hormones: energy level, muscular strength, bone density, sex drive, mental clarity, and the ability to concentrate. The hormone treatment practiced by anti-aging doctors is called

http://www.youtube.com/watch?v=1803KZ7qSes

hormone replacement therapy (HRT). When replacement hormones have the exact same molecular structure as natural human hormones, it is referred to as bio-identical hormone replacement therapy or BHRT. (The 'bio-identical' part of that phrase means that these hormones replicate human hormones rather than being synthetic ones.) Effective and safe hormone therapy requires a thorough understanding of what hormones are and how to balance them.

Hormones are essentially chemical messengers; regulators and modulators. They tell our cells what to do and they tell our bodies what kind of substances to manufacture or when to absorb new energy. They are absolutely necessary for normal physiological function, and need to be in a certain abundance to do their jobs effectively.

Hormone levels reach their peak at the same time we reach the peak of human development and performance, which is usually in our early twenties. After that there is a constant and steady decline. The correlation between the decline in hormones and the decline in human functionality and performance is clear.

http://www.youtube.com/watch?v=S7zWjHCHsH4

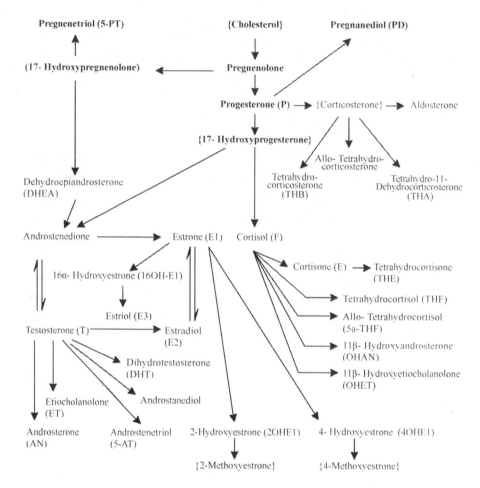

**Biochemistry and Metabolism of Steroid Hormones As Produced
in the Ovaries, Testes and Adrenals**

One theory postulates that aging is actually caused by the decline
of hormones. I don't think this is necessarily true. There is, however,
a clear association between performance and hormone levels.
Whether the decline in hormones causes aging, or aging causes the
decline in hormones is a 'chicken or the egg' conundrum. No one
knows which is first, but the fact remains that hormone levels decline
significantly as we age, and this needs to be addressed just like any
other deficiency.

THIS BRINGS
NEW MEANING
TO THE
PHRASE:
"PUT SOME FUN
IN YOUR LIFE."

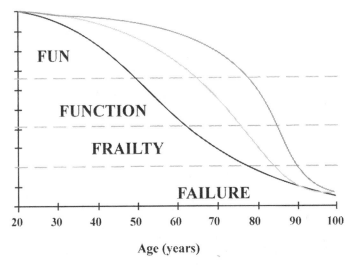

FUN

FUNCTION

FRAILTY

FAILURE

Age (years)

For example, if you have a patient who is diabetic and deficient in insulin, you would treat it by giving them insulin, regardless of whether diabetes caused the drop in insulin or the drop in insulin caused the diabetes. In the same vein, testosterone therapy should be treated with testosterone, regardless of whether aging caused the deficiency or the deficiency caused aging. The same theory holds for a female patient with low estrogen - you would treat with estrogen; and so forth.

HGH AND THE HORMONE-AGING CONNECTION

There are a great many hormones, but the one that has gotten the most attention in recent years - especially in regards to HRT - is human growth hormone, or HGH. This is an essential hormone, produced in the pituitary gland based by signals from the hypothalamus, which lies deep within the brain. HGH is required for your body to grow (hence its name) and for normal organ development until you reach physical maturity, usually around age twenty. Then it starts to de-cline, but remains necessary for maintaining optimal organ function throughout life. HGH also plays a role in controlling the life cycle of cells, although this is not fully understood.

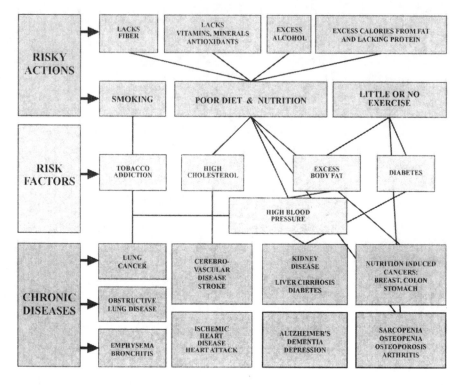

Chronic Diseases and Lifestyle

HGH serves as a good example of what happens to most hormones as they wane (there are a couple of hormones, such as cortisol and insulin, that cause problems by becoming more abundant, but we'll come back to those). For practical purposes, what happens with HGH is what happens with hormones across the board. After you reach your peak - typically somewhere between the ages of twenty and twenty-five - your HGH level declines at a rate of about three percent each year. This rise and subsequent decline corresponds closely to the rise and decline of other hormones. Together they create what I call the 'vitality curve'. This is the arc of energy, health, and maximum functionality during which hormones are most active. This begins almost the day we are born and continues on until we reach capacity in our early twenties, approximately the age when we send men into the armed forces, and also the most ideal reproductive age.

After this maximum functionality declines, things really begin to drop off - usually even more so after age forty.

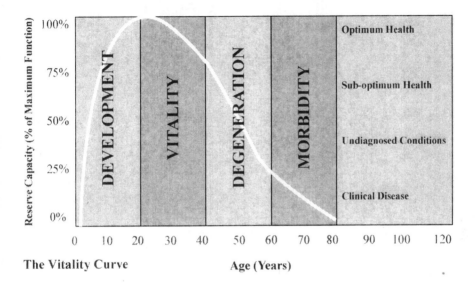

The Vitality Curve

Therefore, under normal conditions, your maximum vitality is going to be between the ages of twenty and forty. After age forty, the soup of your lifestyle and the environment start to take a toll. A degenerative phase sets in. It is silent, but it's happening.

By the time you turn sixty, you are reaching morbidity. All that was silent is no longer silent. Chronic, clinical diseases set in. After optimal health between twenty and twenty-five, most people experience sub-optimal heath until around age forty, with various un-diagnosed conditions after that, and finally, clinical diseases from around sixty onward. Then you die.

QUALITY OF LIFE MARKERS	
1.	Mood
2.	Cognitive Function
3.	Libido
4.	Sexual Performance
5.	Energy
6.	Sleep Quality
7.	Pain Relief
8.	Body Image

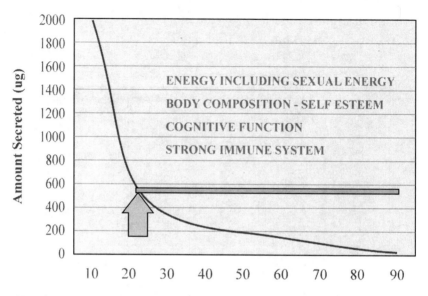

Many hormones including hGH decrease at 1- 3% year.
Hormonal and metabolic balance with exercise is the key to success.

Growth Hormone Decline

What modern medicine focuses on - and where we spend most of our healthcare money - is on that final morbidity stretch of the vitality curve, but it makes far more sense for intervention to take place earlier in the curve. This is what age management and anti-aging medicine is all about. In the anti-aging field we put more resources into the earlier phases of our lives and extend the years of vitality. In terms of practical action, this means extending the years of youthful hormone levels through hormone therapy.

THE REPLACEMENTS

Once we decide to replace depleted hormones, we must understand that this is not a linear, simplistic process. As always, the devil is in the details, and the relationship of hormones to each other and to

http://www.youtube.
com/watch?v=fZaB
By4Kv24

160

other physiological processes is complex. You have to know about these inter-relationships in order to administer hormones and do no harm.

My favorite analogy is that individual hormones are like the instruments in a symphony orchestra. You've got many instruments in the orchestra, but if they are not all in tune, the quality of the music is neither harmonious nor beautiful. You need everything to be in tune for the orchestra to sound great. You have to look at the entire ensemble of hormones to make sure they are in youthful balance; no one hormone is going to be the cure-all answer, just as no one instrument is the orchestra.

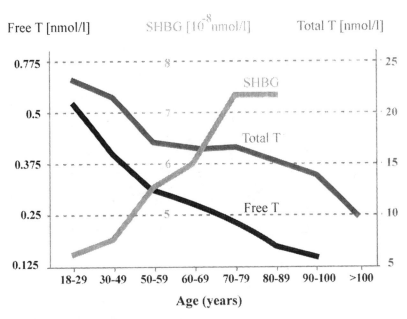

Free T [nmol/l]   SHBG [10^{-8} nmol/l]   Total T [nmol/l]

Age Related Decline in Testicular Function

A lot of people think that HGH is the fountain of youth, but it isn't. It's an important hormone that should be in a reasonably youthful range, but it still has to be in balance with other hormones and can't be treated in isolation. For example, if HGH is not balanced with testosterone it can produce exaggerated androgen effects, because it acts as an activator of testosterone. If people have a deficiency in HGH, we replace it, but it's really just one of many hormones that affect vitality.

I try to figure out what hormones are deficient in a patient by measuring all their hormone levels with blood tests, and then tie that data to how the patient is feeling. Usually we've already recorded a thorough history and general examination, so before I even test for specific hormones, I find that most every response in their examination, most every behavioral symptom and even aesthetic signs I can observe - are tied to the hormone system, or a hormone deficiency.

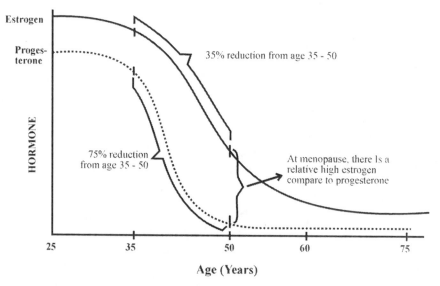

Age Related Decline in Ovarian Function

In terms of looking for deficiencies, I first measure the sex hormones, beginning with testosterone and dihydrotestosterone, estrogen and progesterone for men and women. Beyond measuring just direct levels, I also measure other indicators for additional information about what's going on with the sex hormones. The effects of progesterone and estrogen are meant to balance each other, so they might work against each other, or may ideally complement each other's effects.

For example, estrogen and androgen are designed to cause the body to retain fluid and swell, especially noted in the abdomen and the breasts with estrogen and in the feet and ankles with androgen. Progesterone does just the opposite, acting like a water pill to block the effects of estrogen and androgen, as well as to block the effects of aldosterone, another hormone that promotes water retention and swelling. Estrogen may increase menstrual blood loss whereas progesterone stops the growth of the inner lining of the uterus and thereby reduces menstrual bleeding. Whereas estrogen tends to stimulate the nervous system if uncontrolled and not balanced properly with progesterone, they can cause a woman to be 'nervous'. On the other hand, progesterone has a calming influence on our autonomic nervous system, which is needed for restful sleep and a calmer disposition.

The body is made more feminine by estrogen, and primarily by estradiol. Estrogen is the main reason for the feminine body shape (breasts, widened pelvis, pink/red skin, vaginal lubrication, a healthy female sex drive, the female quality of the voice). They also make menstruation happen because of higher levels present during the early part of the menstrual cycle, causing the inner lining of the uterus to thicken in anticipation of a possible pregnancy. When there is no fertilization or pregnancy, the egg falls dramatically toward the end of the cycle to start the menstrual period. Progesterone complements this by transforming the inner lining of the uterus that has been thickened and preparing for implantation of the fertilized egg, in addition to closing the cervix during pregnancy or during the last phase of the menstrual cycle.

You also have secondary hormones that contribute to the production of the primary sex hormones, and we measure these as well. They include DHEA (dihydroepiandrosterone) and androstenedione, precursors for the sex hormones; and pregnenolone, a precursor for the sex hormones as well as adrenal stress hormones like cortisol. These secondary, precursor hormones are important substrates that convert to more powerful hormones, and if they are deficient your body will try to compensate by pulling from other biochemical pathways. Replacing secondary or precursor hormones stops this pulling from different pathways and helps to balance things out. They also have secondary effects of their own. DHEA, for example, supports the body's immune system and helps protect the body from atherosclerosis.

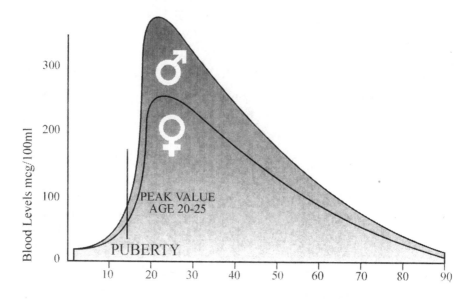

DHEA Levels in Men and Women

After testing HGH, the sex hormones and all their derivatives, comes testing for thyroid function. This is quite important, because thyroid hormones regulate the metabolism of every cell in your body. They regulate energy production, heart rate, blood flow, body warmth, and even the speed of cognitive processes. When you suffer from hypothyroidism - which means an abnormally low level of the thyroid hormone - one typical effect is fatigue. Another is obesity.

A very substantial number of my patients are on thyroid replacement. Hypothyroidism is rampant in our society. I test for that in a number of ways, and again we compare the normal reference range of the thyroid hormone with its functionality in terms of what the patient is experiencing. I then replace it directly or with an iodine supplement, because it is a deficiency in dietary iodine that frequently leads to low thyroid function.

The other hormone levels we measure at RVI include: melatonin, melatonin stimulating hormone, aldosterone, calcitonin, oxytocin, parathormone, vasopressin, insulin-like growth factor (IGF-1), cortisol and glucocorticoids, and insulin.

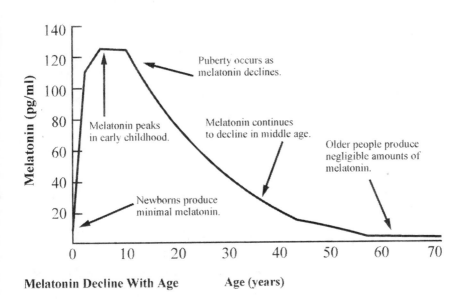

Melatonin Decline With Age

It's All About Balance

We must measure all the hormones, because there is no one master hormone. Every hormone thinks it is the master, but it isn't. It's about getting along with all the other hormones in homeostasis (in balance). About the closest thing we have to a master hormone is pregnenolone, because it is the precursor to many major hormones, especially the sex hormones and the adrenal stress hormones. It is created from cholesterol, so before you give up eating eggs and avocados, remember that substances like testosterone and adrenaline require cholesterol for production. In addition to this very important primary role, pregnenolone also works in the nervous system as a neurohormone and has specific effects in supporting memory. Approximately half of my patients who are on a minimum of 50 mg of pregnenolone a day tell me they have experienced a positive memory improvement.

http://www.youtube.com/watch?v=MJD6e2IUzW8

Hormones, Steroids & Cancer

When it comes to hormone replacement therapy, human growth hormone (HGH) is high on the list, but it is one that comes with controversy because, sadly, it has been misused. For anti-aging purposes we bring HGH levels back to where they were at age 30-40, to about 75 percent of their peak. When HGH is used in excess, however, it behaves like an anabolic steroid. This leads to side effects such as excessive muscle and bone growth.

Like any other substance or medication, if you take too much it becomes harmful. Food is wonderful, but if you eat too much of the wrong things, you get obese and morbidly ill. If you take too much aspirin you can bleed to death. If you take too much vitamin C it can crystallize and cause kidney stones. Anything in excess can be a problem, some things more than others, so why should HGH be any different? Instead of spiking it, we want to maintain it within the range of normal physiology and not exceed that.

Of course, we can debate what normal is. There is a school of thought that says it's normal for nature to allow us to degenerate and become frail and decrepit. If you agree, then an anti-aging regime is not for you.

166

The other school says that maybe, if we improve our hormone balance, we can extend our vitality curve. We are not talking about extending our life spans, because these are set to a maximum of about 120 years. We are talking about extending our years of optimal wellness within our given longevity. We want to extend that vitality - not flood our systems with hormone levels that create steroidal, abnormal growth. That would certainly create a situation that is far from healthy and vital. It would do the exact opposite.

The Consequence of Excess

With HGH, or any hormone, we always want to avoid administering abnormally high amounts. While there is no evidence that clearly demonstrates a cause and effect between human growth hormone and cancer, there are studies that do show an association between the two. Then again, there are studies showing that it protects against cancer. The difference is in the dose. The studies that show a cancer link involve the administration of very high doses. Studies that showed a protection against cancer involved lower doses.

The same high dose situation is what occurs when HGH is labeled a steroid. Technically speaking, HGH is not a steroid. Rather it is an anabolic agent and, as such, stimulates the building up of organs and tissue. It also has androgenic effects, which means it stimulates the development of male sexual characteristics by potentiating the effects of testosterone. So if you have a patient who is on testosterone, and you add growth hormone, they can have the adverse signs and symptoms of too many androgens (male sex hormones) and the traits they produce.

The reason HGH is called a steroid is because of its effects, rather than its molecular structure. Steroids, strictly speaking, are chemical substances with a structure consisting of multiple rings of connected atoms; they typically reduce inflammation. What most people mean by steroids are actually anabolic steroids, synthetic substances related to the male sex hormones (androgens) that promote muscle growth (the anabolic effect).

There are many different types of steroids, from the sex hormones like testosterone, to the adrenal steroids like cortisol, to the glucocorticoids that regulate the metabolism of glucose. Their basic molecular structure is similar, but other side groups are added on that give them different properties and different messaging capabilities. Working as hormonal signalers, they turn on and off different switches in cells.

In addition to natural steroids you have artificial steroids that are synthetically produced. The differences between them are the differences in the side groups related to them, or the different configurations of the molecules: these changes make them more powerful than steroids made by the human body. Indeed, artificially made steroids are very powerful, and do a much stronger job of influencing biological functions than natural steroids.

The synthetic steroids that have received the greatest attention are the androgenic steroids, such as testosterone. These are anabolic steroids. They build tissue, and are the steroids that juice people up. Just like you would expect from somebody with a youthful level of testosterone, these give people something more. They are used by body builders, and for people who want to enhance muscular performance.

This is where you get into trouble with HGH. You can't prescribe it for enhancing physical performance. You can't prescribe it for sore knees. You can only prescribe it for someone who has a diagnosed adult growth hormone deficiency. You can't buy it without a legal medical indication and prescription, that's where the illegality of it comes in.

The lesson here is that hormone replacement therapy must be practiced in a balanced, moderate fashion. If we look at hormones in terms of wellness and vitality, and targeting levels for optimal physiology, the best years are clearly those before the age of 40. People in this age group generally have a more robust level of hormones and are not dying of degenerative, chronic diseases. So the level we target is about the 75th percentile of a man or woman at their peak, somewhere between age 20 and 30, which is a safe yet healthy and youthful physiologic level.

Again, these may not be normal, physiologic levels for a decrepit 70-year old. But why should they be? That's why older people are decrepit. If you want to stay decrepit, just stay at the physiologic hormone levels that are normal for a decrepit 70-year old. But to return us to a vital state in life does not mean abusing hormones to the level of steroids.

THE EXCEPTIONS: HORMONES IN EXCESS

While typically all these hormones need to be restored as they fade away, there are two where the problem lies in the opposite direction: insulin and cortisol. When these are produced in excess, we have a problem - at least until they burn out and need to be replaced along with the rest.

Insulin

First, let's talk about insulin. If I were on a deserted island and wanted just one test to predict how healthy I would be, it would be my fasting insulin level. This is because insulin is the hormone that tells your cells when it's time to absorb sugar from the blood - when it's time to eat. Without any insulin your cells would starve, and without the proper levels of insulin, your metabolism spins out of control.

This is why too much sugar is so unhealthy, because it blows out the insulin mechanisms in your body. When you constantly flood your blood with sugar at levels way beyond what the human diet supplied for millions of years, too much insulin is produced. This leads to insulin insensitivity, which leads to more insulin being produced, greater insensitivity, and so forth. The ultimate result is type 2 diabetes, where there is huge insulin resistance in the cells of the body.

When we detect too much of the insulin hormone, we treat it primarily through diet and exercise. With diet we focus on changing to foods which have a low glycemic load, such as proteins, vegetables, and fruits. Even in the realm of fruits, we have patients consume fruits with low glycemic loads, such as apples and strawberries rather than bananas and raisins. These fruits, like other foods with low glycemic loads, tend to release their sugars more slowly into the blood stream, and so demand less insulin production.

Cortisol

The next hormone I want to control from getting either too high or too low is cortisol, a hormone that helps physiologically in many ways, including increasing blood sugar and blood pressure, fighting inflammation, and enhancing positive moods, energy capacity, resistance to stress and infections, support of the immune system, and positively influencing pain tolerance.

Cortisol helps us adapt to stress by releasing more energy fuel. It's produced when we are under constant low-level stress, the kind that comes from noise, traffic, television, etc. This continuous stress puts a big demand on our adrenal glands to produce increasing amounts of cortisol, which eventually blunts the ability of the adrenal gland to produce more, as if it were used up. Then you start to get too little, and you can't deal with stress at all. You become more susceptible to disease, obesity, and rapid aging.

As with insulin, it's important for us to dampen the production of cortisol before the adrenal glands become exhausted. Too much cortisol also increases insulin resistance and contributes to obesity or weight gain, because cortisol mobilizes energy sources by raising blood sugar over time. It also contributes to chronic inflammation, so you want to bring it down and keep it in a normal range.

In terms of diet, cortisol over-production responds to balanced nutrition just as insulin over-production does. You want to make sure you have enough vitamins and minerals, with special attention to vitamin B complex, vitamin B5 (Pantothenic Acid), vitamin C, zinc, magnesium and eleuthero (formerly known as Siberian ginseng). For high cortisol specifically, you want foods that are high in bioflavonoids or bioflavonoid supplements, or a supplement called phosphorylated serine.

If the adrenal glands have already become too exhausted, I recommend nourishing the adrenals with all of the basic dietary improvements just mentioned, but instead of the bioflavonoids and phosphorylated serine, I prescribe licorice root extract, or just use hydrocortisone to replace the cortisol, until the adrenal glands can recover.

To a remarkable degree, all hormone production responds well to the basics of an anti-aging lifestyle: proper exercise, good sleep, getting outdoors, reducing stress, and consuming a healthy diet. Testosterone requires plenty of protein, for example, and the avoidance of alcohol, caffeine, sugar, tobacco, soft drinks, pastries, milk products, etc. It's also helped by amino acid supplements, just as human growth hormone is helped by glutamine, arginine and lysine supplements, along with a high protein, low carbohydrate diet.

Another approach is to deal with precursors to hormones, which are sometimes called secondary hormones, and to help stimulate the increase in hormones through this indirect path. DHEA is, for example, produced in the peripheral part of the adrenal called the adrenal cortex. You can take this as a supplement that's available in vitamin stores, though I prescribe a sustained release, micronized, compounded version of it for my patients at RVI, to ensure quality and proper, optimal absorption.

DHEA helps to balance cortisol, the main stress hormone. It is also vital in the production of testosterone in women, since they don't have a testicular source. In addition, DHEA has a secondary effect on muscles (which is why athletes take it), on nerotransmitters, and on influencing cognitive function and short-term memroy.

In most cases (regardless of how superb your dietary lifestyle is) hormone deficiencies usually require BHRT (Biomedical Hormone Replacement Therapy). This takes us back full circle, to why we want to correct hormone deficiencies in the first place.

THE IRRITABILITY SYNDROME

The irritability syndrome associated with aging is not inevitable. It's mostly a reaction to the decline in hormones that can be replaced. If you look at it historically, we have been describing the 'male irritability syndrome' for as long as we've been able to describe things. It's become a cliché, from Ebenezer Scrooge right up to the film Grumpy Old Men, but we've never really understood it. Why does it happen? We've pawned it off on everything except biology.

When you look deeper, you begin to understand that the irritability syndrome really does have a biological root, and it's based on what happens to us hormonally.

In men, the grumpy old man syndrome is all about the decline of the androgen, especially the decline of testosterone. Irritability is a classic symptom of testosterone deficiency.

In women the syndrome also occurs with hormonal decline, but the decline is primarily an estrogen deficiency rather than a testosterone deficiency. When women go through menopause, they basically suffer from this. When men go through andropause, the male equivalent, they get the same spectrum of symptoms, namely an irritability syndrome that equals being pissed off at the world. In truth, that's just what it is: being grumpy, pissed off, and unhappy. I have patients go through a list of signs that describe what is happening to them, and the more specific the details of their grumpiness, the worse it is.

No matter how bad it is, however, once you replace what's missing, people feel better. The irritability goes away, and they return to their old selves, feeling perfectly fine and not grumpy or pissed off, because they've addressed the biological root of the problem. The results are tremendous in terms of the influence on a person's life. Let's face it, when you're irritable all the time it affects every dimension of your day, from social relationships with friends, family, and significant others, to work relationships with clients, colleagues, and co-workers. It deteriorates your harmonious relationship with the whole world and it becomes a self-fulfilling syndrome.

In almost every case of the irritability syndrome, there is a hormonal basis. In some cases this is the first sign of hormonal decline, and in many cases a lab test is little more than a technicality, because the diagnosis is so obvious. In some patients, it is the paramount issue, much more important to them personally than the loss of libido or loss of muscle mass. Their daily life is being messed up because they are so damn cranky all the time. It's a critical factor for them.

One interesting question is whether the irritability syndrome is inevitable with aging. Certainly there are cases of people considered saintly in their old age, an elderly priest or monk with tremendous beneficence. Just think of Mother Teresa: kind, gentle, loving, etc. Is there a biochemical basis to this, or have these people trained themselves to transcend the syndrome?

First, I would say that saintly people are more the exception than the rule. You don't see a large population of beneficent people walking around the planet; that's why they are canonized as saints. The real question is why these people are like this. Unfortunately, this has not yet been studied; we have not measured hormone levels of beneficent people and compared them to those of the general population. We can really only postulate.

Perhaps these so-called beneficent people are as grumpy and irritable as the rest of us, but really good actors. Perhaps they know how to, when necessary, put a muzzle on the syndrome and appear calm to rest of the world. Another possibility is that they have some kind of compensation through their neural transmitters, perhaps higher than average serotonin levels for example, or very low dopamine levels, so they are walking around like pseudo zombies, very calm and very beneficent, even though they have hormonal declines.

Like anything else, you can't compartmentalize everything. Just because someone isn't irritable doesn't mean they don't have a hormone deficiency. There may be other things going on, like a regimen of meditation. Indeed, meditation and other Eastern disciplines have demonstrable biochemical effects, including changes to neurotransmitters that can influence mood and affect personality. These people are going to behave differently; they are going to feel differently, and you're going to sense that they are different.

Spirituality, prayer, and meditation - all of these things have calming influences on personality. No matter what's going on under the surface, these practices enable people to appear and behave more serenely. Many people consider this an integral part of their lives, and for them it is beneficial. It's not mandatory for our protocol, but is certainly worth mentioning.

PREVENTING FRAILTY

The beginning of the end for most elderly people is when they start to get frail. The fact is that most frailty is preventable and very easily treatable, with testosterone as well as human growth hormone (HGH), combined with exercise and diet. It is just basic hormonal replacement therapy (HRT).

For the record, gerontologists typically don't advocate this. They don't believe in hormone replacement therapy for elderly people because they largely believe that the damage is already done. They think you can be old and decrepit and frail, but consider the fact that your testosterone is low to be irrelevant. They believe it's too late.

http.//www.youtube
com/watch?v=Rqrj
rgr8f8l

Fortunately, there are studies now being funded by the National Institute on Aging that will prove the value of BHRT, but unfortunately the amount being spent to study BHRT is miniscule. This lack of attention toward preventing frailty is a big weakness of our national health system. We spend eighty percent of all medical dollars on the last few years of life, with very little of this money going toward studying how to prevent the frailty of old age.

This is why I'm not a gerontologist. I don't want to treat people for the diseases of aging. I want to prevent those diseases and do whatever I can to build the elderly up to fight them and avoid frailty. I want old people to lead vital, active lives.

Sometimes, it is too late. For someone who is very old and has a lot of serious, chronic diseases, it's late in the game and there is a limit to what can be done. If they already have advanced conditions, anti-aging doctors don't have any magic in their toolboxes to bring them back, but we can certainly help somebody delay or avoid getting there.

Another piece of good news is that it's relatively inexpensive. A little testosterone, some dietary changes, a few yoga classes, some walking, a few weights - these are modest costs. It does not take wealth to practice anti-aging. The only thing that is expensive is human growth hormone, partly because it's not covered by insurance as other supplements are. Most insurance will cover testosterone deficiency, for example, if that is the diagnosis.

When it comes to modifying your diet, it's true that it's more expensive to buy and eat organic food, but with an anti-aging diet you are going to eat less and tend to eat more often at home instead of eating out, so the expense will balance out. The trade is quality versus quantity, wholesome versus processed. It doesn't need to be expensive to implement either change, and you don't need a fancy gym or a personal trainer. You can do this.

The basic items needed for a healthy anti-aging program probably cost less than what you spend on other frivolities. Testosterone, even if you are paying cash, will probably cost no more than $30 or $40 a month. HGH, by comparison, will cost anywhere from $350 to $1200 a month, but even with HGH, there are less expensive medications. Sermorelin, which is a growth hormone releasing hormone (GHRH), or HGH secretagogues (human growth hormone stimulators) work better in younger adults and cost closer to $150 a month.

When we correct hormone imbalances and restore those that are deficient, frailty can definitely be prevented, improved or even reversed, with an enormous benefit to society as a whole and in particular to the geriatric population, which is growing exponentially.

Participating in an anti-aging medicine program means not becoming one of those frail people. Bio-identical hormone replacement therapy (BHRT) is one of the great tools in the anti-aging arsenal. We restore what's missing - or dampen what's in excess - and then complete the recovery process with diet, exercise, sleep, and stress management.

THE AESTHETICS
OF YOUTH

CHAPTER 10

Our goal in anti-aging medicine is to help you be the best, healthiest, strongest, most energetic you possible. Not only do you want to be the best version of you, but you want to look your best, too. Sometimes that involves a little extra help. Fortunately, technology has advanced considerably and little 'fixes' can be made without extreme costs or downtime.

http://www.youtube.com/watch?v=Q0yfzGp-VUs

A LITTLE EXTRA HELP

More and more anti-aging doctors also practice some cosmetic procedures, especially the non-invasive or minimally invasive methods used to sculpt a patient's face or body.

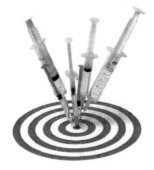

It's become fairly standard to use injectable fillers: collagen stimulators, muscle paralyzing agents, chemical peels, and lasers, to enhance the face. The in-vogue treatment for the body and the face is to transfer fat. This involves moving fat from one part of the body where you have extra to spare, to somewhere else where there is depleted volume.

Effectively treating a patient cosmetically requires a thorough understanding of facial anatomy and an understanding of how men and women age differently. People lose muscle mass, bone mass, and fat mass, and you have to know what has contributed to the age-related changes. You want to look more like a Rembrandt than a Picasso when you're finished, and you certainly never want your patients to look 'done'. Most of what we find attractive in others is subliminal, and my goal is to optimize those unique features for each patient.

BEHIND MEN'S ATTRACTIVENESS

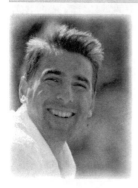

- Facial attractiveness results from a mixture of symmetry and averageness of traits
- Overhanging horizontal brow with minimal arch
- Angular facial features
- Deeper set eyes and a larger nose which makes eyes appear closer set
- Wider nose and mouth
- Larger lower face and jaw
- Squared lower face with muscular masticator muscles
- Waist-to-hip ratio (WHR)

BEHIND WOMEN'S ATTRACTIVENESS

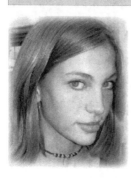

- Facial attractiveness results from a mixture of symmetry and averageness of traits
- High forehead and cheekbones
- Small nose and chin
- Wide eyes
- Full lips
- Thin eyebrows
- Thick hair
- A low Waist Hip ratio

Returning the face and body to a more youthful and attractive appearance depends on a deep understanding of the aging process. This book is not about cosmetic surgery, but it is nonetheless important to understand some of the treatment options available. This is especially true for making the face look younger. The aesthetic training and sensibility of a doctor is crucial.

While wrinkles are a key component of the aging appearance, the localized and or generalized loss of facial volume is the paramount indicator of aging, and with it the sagging of skin. I'm meticulous about carefully examining the faces of my patients and their anatomy, and looking closely at where their age shows most. When you and looking closely at where their age shows most. When you plan treatment this way there is a much higher chance of achieving natural looking, youthful improvement.

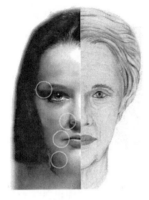

Restoring volume is the key to achieving a youthful look, so the question of which volume-restoring material or technique to use becomes crucial. Some anti-aging doctors and cosmetic surgeons use body fat to restore facial volume. Enriching fat removed for transfer with platelet-rich plasma derived from the patient's blood and/or stem cells is a current cutting edge technique that has really improved results. My approach is to select a volume-enhancing treatment that best addresses each patient's unique issues, anatomy, biology, and budget. Some patients are seeking short-term and less expensive solutions, while others are looking for long-term solutions. Some want a dramatic, immediate change, while others desire a more subtle and gradual improvement.

THE FACIAL AGING PROCESS

PREMATURE AGING
- Sun exposure
- Smoking
- Chronological aging
- Genetics

HEALTHY SKIN
- Smooth
- Soft
- Firm
- Glowing,
- Even pigmentation

- Clear of blemishes and vascular lesions
- Plump with natural moisture

- Adequate subcutaneous collagen and fat to provide youthful contour and complexion

THE COLLAGEN CONNECTION

To satisfy the disparate requirements of different patients, I select the appropriate injectable fillers, and/or collagen stimulators, which are either short or long-term acting, to fit each patient's situation and provide the desired outcome. While many of these volume-enhancing materials are not fat, they simulate fat volume and, more importantly, encourage the production of collagen. Collagen is a protein that acts as the foundation matrix for connective tissue. It's like scaffolding; it holds your soft tissue together, and gives it structural rigidity.

There is a little bit of collagen in all fat, mostly in fibrils intertwined with fat globules that keep them in place, but most collagen is in skin. It lies in the connective tissue just below the skin, as well as in the muscle below that. When you lose collagen you immediately lose the foundational, structural support of the connective tissue, which results in a sagging, drooping look. Trying to keep your skin looking young without collagen is like trying to build a house without a foundation; it won't sit very well.

Injectable fillers offer the key advantages of instant results and no down time. They may also be the only alternative for some patients who are 'fat challenged'. Some of the patients I see in Beverly Hills are way too thin to be good candidates for fat transfer. Each patient has unique needs, so I go over all the options with them, to come up with the best solutions for each individual. These include the products which stimulate collagen and make a patient's own skin thicken itself.

DEALING WITH WRINKLES

The other significant sign of facial aging, beyond loss of volume, is the appearance of wrinkles. To understand how to reduce or eliminate them, however, you have to first understand that there are different types of wrinkles and different types of anatomies under those wrinkles. You have to understand what causes wrinkles in order to deal with them.

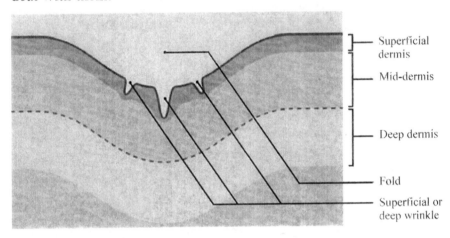

There are actually three types of wrinkles. The first type is caused by aging skin, including exposure to the environment (especially ultraviolet light from the sun or tanning booths), and smoking. There are also wrinkles that result from loss of facial fat volume, muscle, and bone loss. The third type of wrinkle is the result of muscular contraction.

If the wrinkle is the result of skin aging and/or exposure, and the patient has an adequate amount of fat volume with good muscular and bone structure, the treatments are going to be skin deep, literally. I would work on the surface of the skin or close to it, to achieve desired results.

These kinds of wrinkles also respond very well to chemical peels and lasers. They help resurface the skin, minimizing wrinkles while evening out skin tones and pigments. These treatments can also help tighten the skin and build collagen (but in a different way than fillers). The best skin resurfacing lasers are called ablative lasers, which resurface the skin so it can rebuild itself in a smoother, more youthful looking way.

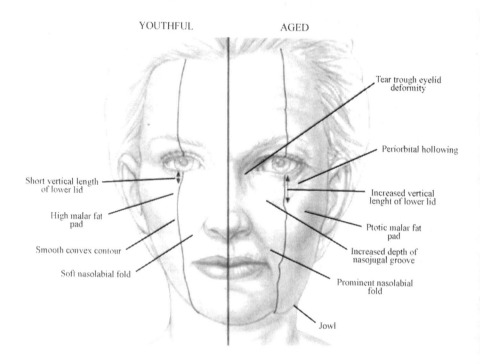

Unlike the skin resurfacing lasers we used just seven or eight years ago (which vaporized the entire skin surface off), the lasers used now are 'pixilated' or fractional. This means that they vaporize little columns of damaged skin within the healthy skin, like tiny polka dots on the surface. This promotes rapid healing and minimizes risk. The important thing is to what depth you go. Obviously, the deeper the wrinkle or higher the degree of skin laxity, the more depth you need to penetrate. but you have to be careful not to go too deep, because healthy tissue is at risk of being destroyed.

There are other types of lasers, each with its own unique benefits. Skin tightening lasers work below the surface, in the middle and lower dermis, to build collagen. Pigment directed lasers, which usually work on all the layers of the skin, attack pigment related issues. An example of a pigment directed laser is the IPL, or intense pulsed light device. Although technically not a laser, IPL is used to even out brown or red pigment, shrink pore size, improve the luster/reflectivity of the skin and improve the very finest of wrinkles. It can also be used to treat some cases of acne and rosacea.

The technology behind these lasers has advanced to the point where they're much safer than those of the past. There is little or no pain, and recovery time is minimal if any. There is no such thing as zero risk, but when these treatments are administered correctly, the risks are very low.

Deeper Wrinkles

Lasers don't help, however, with wrinkles that are a result of a patient's depleted volume. This loss of volume creates deeper wrinkles, and the only way to really deal with them is to bring back more volume, as we discussed above. The treatment is deeper, using fat transfer or some type of deep synthetic filler injection.

Think of this type of wrinkle like the skin of a raisin. If you inject water into the middle of the raisin, it plumps up and becomes smoother - more like a grape. If, however, you inject the water just under the surface of the raisin's skin, it's going to look like a raisin with a little fattened area of skin. It's not going to look like a grape. It's the same thing with the face. You have to carefully analyze the structure of the patient's face, then choose treatments that work to restore the overall volume.

Muscle contractions also cause skin to wrinkle. To deal with this third type of wrinkle, I would again examine the muscle groups within the face. I then select a neural toxin to relax certain muscles in key places.

The treatment usually used is called Botox®, although there are a handful of other treatments such as Dysport® and Xeomin® that are used as well. When done correctly, the result is a smoother, refreshed look, not an expressionless face.

We address wrinkles, like other aspects of anti-aging, with multiple, customizable approaches. Deeper wrinkles typically require some kind of injectable filler or collagen stimulator suitable for deep volume collagen building, or we may use a fat transfer. More super-ficial wrinkles require fillers that can be used on the surface of the skin, such as hyaluronic acid fillers like Restylane®, Perlane®, Juvederm® and Belotero® or others like Radiesse® or Artefill®. I might resurface the skin with lasers or a chemical peel. Many patients have all three types of wrinkles or a combination thereof. Doctors must carefully evaluate each patient to provide the combination of remedies that will garner the best results.

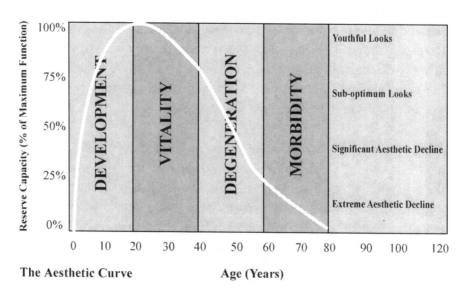

The Aesthetic Curve   Age (Years)

Additionally, successful treatment involves making patients feel as comfortable as possible. You can do the best work in the world and your results can be fantastic, but if the patient has pain, they won't like it and won't follow through on their commitment to the larger anti-aging program. Pain is a very big deal, especially when pursuing an aesthetic goal.

DETOXIFYING YOUR ENVIRONMENT

CHAPTER 11

Among the various controversies surrounding anti-aging medicine and the struggle to live a healthier, less damaging lifestyle is the issue of environmental pollution. Pollutants are typically silent, invisible, and take a long time to manifest their effects. Those who scoff at setting environmental standards argue that we exaggerate their effects.

It is my opinion, however, that the degraded quality of our water, air, soil, and even our light combine to slowly, inexorably wear down the human body - eventually decimating our cellular structure - leading to chronic disease. Once people become keenly aware of this, they will make whatever lifestyle environmental changes they are capable of, to improve the environ-

http://www.youtube.com/watch?v=2lzTnFayY9s

ment in which they spend their days, and move from the obvious improvements of better diet, exercise, improved sleep, and less stress, to the more subtle aspect of removing toxins from their daily lives.

WATER, WATER, EVERYWHERE

You consume more water than any other substance. You put it into your body every single day, but do you think about what's in it? Could there be something in it that affects your wellness, or even your lifespan? People need to think about that because there are impurities in some water that are not good for you.

Additives

Fluoride is one example of an additive commonly found in tap water. It was originally introduced to water sources after WW2 as a way to reduce tooth decay. The population then was considerably less aware of oral hygiene than we are today. Fluoridation, along with bromides in our baked goods, has contributed to an epidemic of iodine deficiency. Iodine deficiency can be a cause of sub-clinical hypothyroidism, which may contribute to the development of obesity. We don't need fluoridated water and I don't recommend it, and yet most municipal water supplies are fluoridated. This is just one example of unhealthy additives in our water supply.

One solution is to buy water, but even here there's a double-edge sword. Most water for sale comes in plastic bottles. We now know that the chemicals in plastic bottles leech out into the water and are toxic. While it is only a few parts per billion, the potential effect is significant. Much of the research is fairly new, and we don't understand the full impact yet. How will this affect cancer rates or fertility rates? Will it cause chromosome damage? The evidence now clearly supports the fact that we are witnessing poisoning on a grand scale.

http://water.epa.gov/drink/local/

Glass bottles are the way to go, but they are often hard to find, are heavier to carry, and require a commitment that some people are not willing to make. The good news is that glass bottles don't sit for generations in landfills, nor do they add any toxic residue to your environment. Consider the possibilities.

Where Does It Come From, and How Is It Stored?

The next consideration is the source. Is spring water better than filtered water? Spring water can be very good, but check the source. Make sure you're not drinking water that is high in salt. Also look for water that is more alkaline than acid. Alkalinity protects the body from free-radical oxidation, a major contributor to cellular inflammation, aging, and increased risk for chronic disease. Aside from that, most spring water is probably fine, as is most mineral water. Mineral water is a wonderful source of - you guessed it - minerals. It also tastes better to a lot of people, and that is important when you're trying to drink at least two liters of water daily.

Having said that, it's not clear whether there is a significant benefit from spring water compared to filtered water. If it's clear and pure, then filtered water is probably okay. Think about how our ancestors got their water. They took from natural water sources, with a learned appreciation for moving water over still water. Fewer people probably got sick or died from drinking moving water, without knowing in the earliest days that water in motion undergoes a simple form of filtration, with the sediment filtered out.

As far as the volume of water you should drink, there are various formulas. The standard is half an ounce per pound of body weight, which translates into daily consumption of one hundred ounces, or about three liters, for a two hundred pound man. Did our ancestors really drink that much? It is impossible to say. We can only assume that they were in touch with their natural body signals, and hence to real thirst, and that the sources of their water were natural. When planning how much you should drink, keep in mind that the body draws water from a variety of sources, including the food we eat and from other liquids.

If you're not living near a spring - and few people are - your best bet is water in glass bottles. You also can install a good home filtration system for your tap water. In addition to reducing impurities and harmful additives, these systems can also alkalinize the water.

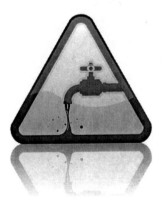

Water Quality
1,200,000,000,000 gallons of:
- *Untreated sewage*
- *Storm water*
- *Industrial toxic materials with radioactive particles are discharged into American waters every year causing 1 in 10 Americans to fall sick each year!*
- **Are YOU in danger?**

Almost 20 million Americans fall ill each year from drinking water contaminated with parasites, bacteria or viruses according to a study published last year in the Scientific Journal of Environmental Contamination and Toxicology.

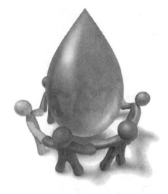

There are 77,000 chemicals being produced every year. Many of them end up in our waters, without any color, scent or taste and then accumulate inside our bodies.

The average person in New York has 540 toxic chemicals in their body and the average baby is now born with 229 chemicals in their blood and organs.

THE AIR WE BREATHE

http://www.youtube.com/watch?v=OOdO-xnOdKs

Air pollution has been recognized for many decades as a cause of illness and disease. Air pollution in cities is mainly caused by the burning of fossil fuels and industrial emissions. It has become so bad that, in the United States at least, regulations have been implemented with some effect. As a result of new regulations, air quality in many American cities - most notably Los Angeles and New York - has improved in recent years.

We still have a long way to go, however, and there is really not a lot you can do to improve your ambient air quality beyond moving to the countryside, relocating to a new city, or living in a different area of the city where you now reside, but of course you can only do what is feasible given your economic situation and your lifestyle.

There are a number of devices you can buy to filter the air in your home or office. The most effective add negative ions to your immediate atmosphere, air that is rich in negative ions - negatively charged molecules - and better for you than air which is poor in such ions, though scientists don't exactly know why. Some studies suggest that negative ions, once they reach the bloodstream, increase our levels of serotonin, combating depression, relieving stress, and boosting energy. Others surmise that inhaling negative ions increases the flow of oxygen to the brain - enhancing mental alertness and cognitive capabilities.

Regardless of how they work, the anecdotal evidence that negative ions have a positive effect is overwhelming. They are created in nature as air molecules break apart due to sunlight, radiation, and the movement of air and water. They are abundant near the beach and waterfalls, in windswept mountain settings, and after a spring thunderstorm - all settings where people report enhanced or elevated moods.

Studies at Columbia University have shown that negative-ion generators for home use are as effective in mood elevation as anti-depressant medication. Therefore, I recommend acquiring a device that can add negative ions to the atmosphere in your rooms. If possible, get a device for both your home and office. You can also seek environments with higher concentrations of negative ions. In both cases you are not only getting more of the negatively charged particles, but cleaner air.

Pollutants are typically bound up by such ions. The quantity of negative ions is depleted by pollutants. This is another reason polluted air is less than optimal, and another reason to generate and seek out more of the ions that make you feel young and more vibrant. And, by the way, stay far away from cigarette smoke.

LET THERE BE LIGHT

The final thing you can improve is the lighting in your environment. It is very important that we expose ourselves to what is called full-spectrum light. Most people don't get enough and the consequences range from inadequate levels of Vitamin D (which is produced by exposure to natural light) to outright depression. This can be witnessed by visiting the Northeast during the winter months. Half the population is walking around depressed and a lot of that has to do with reduced light exposure. Research from countries with deep winters, such as Scandinavia, indicates much higher levels of suicidal and clinical depression in winter months.

Most of us spend too much time under artificial light. We often get up before the sun has risen. We go to offices full of fluorescent lighting, and if we're lucky, get to see the sun for a few moments at the end of our day. That's why I always tell my patients to leave the office during their lunch hour, if only to get outside and walk around the block a couple of times.

Don't forget that in terms of evolution, it's only been a very short while since we've been removed from at least indirect exposure to natural light for most of the day. Our biology is built on such exposure and linked to the rhythms of light and darkness. This is just another example of how disrespect for our biology is causing havoc.

From my own observations of patients, I have found that people who do not have regular exposure to ambient, full-spectrum lighting are never as well as people who do. There hasn't been a lot of research, but the studies completed so far overwhelmingly support this idea. Laboratory rats that lived exclusively under fluorescent lighting, for example, lived only half as long as rats that lived under natural lighting. Fluorescent lighting also increased their rates of cancer. In humans, fluorescent lighting (which has a high-frequency and emits radio frequencies, among other things) has been linked to attention deficit disorders and fatigue, as well as hyperactivity and irritability in children. Switching to full, natural light spectrums reduces these symptoms.

YOU CAN MANAGE YOUR ENVIRONMENT

Anti-aging doctors and other practitioners devoted to enabling others to live their best life truly enjoy witnessing the progress people make when they change their lifestyles, even if the change seems 'almost too easy', such as getting some sunlight or changing out their light bulbs. I tell patients that even if they can't get out as often as they'd like, they should at least get some full-spectrum lighting and install it. It's not quite as relaxing as going for a walk, and it isn't going to mitigate stress as much, but it definitely will help.

Cleaning up your immediate environment comes down to the basic triad of breathing clean air, drinking clean water, and living under natural light during the normal light cycles. You need a good two to three liters of clean water each day. You need clean, fresh air that includes negative ions. Clean your air with the highest-quality air filters you can find, and make sure you are exposed to as much full-spectrum light as possible, even if that means installing special bulbs that replicate the natural spectrum.

I bring these issues and strategies to the attention of all my RVI patients. I tell them, "Go to the beach or someplace where there is no smog, and just close your eyes and breathe the air. Then go downtown in the middle of rush hour, close your eyes and breathe the air. Then tell me how you feel in one place versus the other."

You will quickly realize that our environment has a huge impact on our physical health, as well as our psyche. By being aware of our environment, we can strive to create spaces and routines that benefit our health.

NEUROTRANSMITTERS AND THE BRAIN

CHAPTER 12

The human brain is the big controller. It's the most powerful organ in the body. Its ability to think cognitively and feel emotions is what makes us human. It is the cerebral cortex that sets us apart from other creatures, and we have to respect the thing that makes us special.

There are two issues with the brain related to anti-aging. First is the issue of neural growth. There is some debate as to whether new neurons can be created throughout our lifespan. You may have a finite number of brain cells, and that number keeps decreasing as you get older, but with one hundred billion brain cells to start with there is a huge reserve. In fact, most of

http://www.youtube.com/watch?v=p4kPGNkYbrE

us use only a small part of our neural capacity. Stem cell therapies may eventually get us there, but we currently can create new pathways within the brain, and new circuitry from existing neurons; doing so is extremely important to the health and vitality of our brains. That's what happens when you learn.

Our ability to remain lucid and intelligent as we age first depends on preserving the brain cells we have and then stimulating them to create new pathways. You want to do everything you can to not lose your brain cells too fast - which means staying away from things that kill them, while regenerating the circuits through mental activity. Individuals who maintain vital intellectual lives tend to avoid dementia and live longer.

The second issue with the brain in terms of anti-aging is neurotransmitter balance. This is one of the key things I check for when I take patient histories. Based on this information I can assess what the issues are, and whether they're related to one of the four dominant neurotransmitters: dopamine, acetylcholine, GABA, serotonin, or a combination of the four.

We can then focus on improving deficiencies. I work on correcting the primary deficiency first, and once that's been tackled, we go on to the secondary and then tertiary deficiency, then retest.

Neurotransmitter balance is essential because it underlies how we function. Each neurotransmitter controls certain behaviors and functions, and their deficiencies produce symptoms. Once you get an understanding of the symptoms involved in neurotransmitter imbalances, you have a roadmap for diagnosis and can do something to modify it.

THE BRAIN BALANCE NATURE (ASSESSMENT)

Function: brain energy, motivation / creativity
Deficiency symptoms:

- Sugar / caffeine cravings
- Fatigue
- Lightheadedness
- Weight gain
- Diminished libido
- Low energy
- Memory changes
- Decreased motivation
- Lack of initiative
- Sleep disturbance
- Increased alcohol and drug consumption

Function: brain rhythm, or calm
Deficiency Symptoms:

- Carbohydrate craving
- Trembling, twitching
- Anxiety
- Insomnia
- Hyperventilation
- Palpitations, fast pulse
- Cold or clammy hands
- Ringing in ear, lump in throat, butterflies in stomach
- High blood pressure
- IBS / GI disorders
- Memory changes
- Disorganization
- Depression / Isolation

Function: Brain speed / mental acuity
Deficiency Symptoms:

- Fat cravings
- Weight gain
- Memory lapses
- Difficulty concentrating
- Dry mouth
- Urinary frequency
- Mood changes
- Dyslexia
- Agitation
- Anxiety

SEROTONIN

Function: Brain balance, or mood

Deficiency Symptoms:

- Salt cravings
- Backache or muscle aches
- Neck pain
- Headache

- Shortness of breath
- Insomnia
- PMS
- Sexual Dysfunction

- Weight Gain
- Increased alcohol or nicotine use
- Agitation / anxiety

In order to identify both your dominant nature and possible biochemical deficiencies, you can take a simple test in the privacy of your own home. This twenty-minute profile, which I call the Rejuvalife Nature Assessment, identifies your dominant brain chemistry by both examining physical symptoms and evaluating the psychological dimensions of temperament, type, and personality. The assessment can also reveal the early stages of a brain biochemical deficiency. This will explain the subtle symptoms you experience when you don't feel quite right? The results of these tests then become the guide for many of your health-related issues.

KEEPING IT BALANCED

To understand these neurochemical imbalances, look at it this way, each of us has a certain dominant nature that we are born with and will probably have all our lives, but the dominant traits are relative, not absolute. Your nature relates to your brain chemistry. You may naturally have a somewhat dominant dopamine nature, with relative deficiencies in other neurotransmitters. The goal is to have as much balance as possible. Once the level is balanced, it creates energy, harmony, speed, and happiness. When it's all working together like the symphony example given earlier, that's the ideal state.

Most of us don't have the ideal balance. We have a dominant nature and then minor deficiencies. Many of the patients I see have moderate or severe deficiencies. The spectrum runs from a patient with minimal cognitive

http://www.youtube com/watch?v=jIRN 9xXBidU

impairment, to those on their way to Alzheimer's, or patients who feel just a little off compared to those who are clinically depressed. The key is to identify the nature of each person, determine if there are any real deficiencies, and then promote better balance.

A normal balance and healthy range of hormones contributes to better cognitive function, as will a good diet and adequate exercise. I first determine which neurotransmitter levels are low, and then address them through diet, supplements, hormone replacement, and lifestyle changes. Pharmaceutical solutions should only be used as a final resort, or sometimes a temporary strategy on the road to a more long term solution.

Modifying Neurotransmitters

How do we modify neurotransmitters? Let's look at the example of dopamine. This is a neurotransmitter essential for mental energy and motivation. In the simplest sense, you don't feel like doing anything if you don't have enough dopamine. You feel useless. We want these levels to be high, so first I make sure that if the patient uses medications, they use dopamine-friendly medications, meaning those that help support dopamine.

Next I look at the patient's diet, and explore the dietary options that can help them. In the case of dopamine, for example, L-tyrosine and L-phenylalanine are very important. I recommend foods that are high in the amino acids tyrosine and phenylalanine such as lean meats and dairy, and we try to work that into their diets. Next, we discuss which vitamins and supplements boost dopamine levels. I walk the patient through the natural hormones that can help, and I may prescribe hormone replacement therapy. Once a patient is on this regimen, they quickly notice that they feel much better. They have fewer cravings, more energy, better success with weight loss, and so forth. Why? Because the brain rules. Once we deal with the brain, everything flows from there.

NEUROTRANSMITTERS:
WHAT THEY'RE DESIGNED TO DO

This brings us to the neurotransmitters themselves, and a quick overview of their brain functions.

Brain cells communicate with each other by firing off electrical discharges, which travel along the axon of the cell. The next cell picks up this spark with tiny receptors, called dendrites. The places where the brain cells' branching networks of axons and dendrites connect to each other are called the synapses. What actually crosses the 'synaptic gap' between the cells are the chemicals known as neurotransmitters.

This is where the brain's complexity starts to add up. There may be as many as ten thousand synaptic connections between one neuron and other neurons in the brain. There are also more than fifty types of neurotransmitters identified, though we are concerned here with only the four dominant ones. Each of these is important for a type of neural activity that is relevant to our experience and functionality as humans.

Dopamine

Dopamine is the 'get-up-and-go' transmitter. It's the one that makes you feel like you've got the mental energy to do what you need to do. People who have high dopamine levels have good brain energy. It's not about mental processing speed; it's about the energy you bring. People with low dopamine are tired, lethargic, and moody. They are frequently overweight because they have a tendency to use sugar and simple carbohydrates to get energy. For the same reason they have a tendency to use more stimulants, such as caffeine. They have a tendency to abuse drugs and alcohol a little more than average. They are often insomniacs and may also suffer from impotence. In general, people with low dopamine have a low brain energy spectrum, which is significant because you can't really function well if your brain doesn't have enough energy.

Dopamine also plays a big role in behavior, especially in the areas of motivation, punishment, and reward. It also has a big part in attention, working memory, and learning. Dopamine is believed to contribute to learning by making the connection between behavior and reward. Basically, dopamine provides the feelings of enjoyment and reinforcement that motivate a person to perform certain activities. In terms of the more obvious pleasures in life, it is released by such experiences as eating food and having sex. Some drugs, such as cocaine and nicotine, are associated with their ability to increase dopamine levels.

A low dopamine level has other consequences. Dopamine plays an important function in voluntary movement, so really low levels can lead to the loss of smooth, controlled movement (a.k.a. Parkinson's disease). Low dopamine can also lead to reduced memory, attention deficit disorders, antisocial behavior, and apathy.

For the most part, however, when you've got low dopamine you've got a deficit of energy, motivation, creativity, and quality sleep. A typical story is a patient who is tired, has no sex drive, has carbohydrate cravings, and a poor diet. Indeed, most of the negative conditions that happen to people with low dopamine are connected with being generally overweight - high cholesterol, high blood pressure, insulin insensitivity, etc.

GABA

Just as the energy provided by dopamine is essential for brain function, the rhythm of your brain is equally vital. GABA, short for gamma amino butyric acid, is the neurotransmitter that controls your brain rhythms and levels of neuronal excitability throughout the central nervous system. It acts like a modulator and a balancer; it basically makes people calm. It also acts like a traffic cop that helps control the overall biochemistry of the brain.

Increased levels of GABA typically have a relaxing, anti-anxiety effect. People with high levels of GABA feel peaceful. Those with low levels tend to feel more anxiety. They experience lower pain thresholds and tend to experience chronic bone or back pain. They are typically quite irritable. They often have trouble sleeping and making decisions. They have body pains. Because their brain waves are not in balance, they can experience other imbalances, such as irregular heartbeat. Mostly they have trouble getting things in order. They generally have trouble with relationships and often can't keep a job.

GABA is also responsible for the regulation of muscle tone, so spastic behavior occurs when GABA levels are imbalanced; and increased levels have anti-convulsive effects. The main thing, however, is that GABA reduces the neural excitation that is associated with restlessness, irritability, insomnia, and even seizures. Barbiturates, for example, induce relaxation by stimulating GABA receptors in neurons. The effects of low GABA are seen in excessive worry, panic, poor sleep, high cortisol levels, mood swings, strained personal relationships, and self-medicating to avoid stress.

Acetylcholine

Whereas dopamine was the neurotransmitter for brain energy, and GABA is about brain rhythm, acetylcholine is the neurotransmitter for brain speed. Like the RAM in a computer, it's all about memory access, cognition, speed of processing, and improving your IQ. If you want to improve your ability to learn or increase reading speed, acetylcholine is what you need.

Now, a lot of how to be smart is what we've already talked about in terms of lifestyle, because you need that healthy, biochemical foundation to be smart; but more specifically, you need to boost the neurotransmitters associated with being smart. That's the bottom line - even if you have a lot of RAM, you still won't be able to do very well if your other brain chemicals are out of whack. They all have to work together and be in balance. The concept of balance cannot be stressed enough.

Acetylcholine helps the brain run faster. It affects the elasticity of our brains, which really means our ability to learn and create new memories. It influences our state of arousal and enhances sensory perception. This helps us sustain attention and process input. In essence, it enhances our synaptic transmissions, and its absence is associated with Alzheimer's and dementia.

Acetylcholine has other functions, as well. It plays an important role in producing REM sleep, and affects the cardiovascular system (acting as a vasodilator), the gastrointestinal system, the urinary tracts, and the respiratory system. Its main role in anti-aging, however, is in cognition.

Low levels of acetylcholine lead to all the symptoms that Baby Boomers fear most: forgetfulness, difficulty finding the right words to say, difficulty paying attention, difficulty thinking, short-term memory loss and disorientation; in other words, difficulty with the thinking required for everyday living.

Serotonin

Serotonin is important for many things, but its main role comes down to one word: happiness. It is known as the 'happiness hormone' even though it is not a hormone, because people who have high serotonin levels are happy. People who have less serotonin are less happy. The manifestation of this deficiency is unhappiness, whatever that is for you. It may mean being grumpy and agitated, to having headaches and a stiff neck. People who suffer from a lack of serotonin have a tendency towards depression, which can range from low level to serious.

How or why serotonin contributes to feelings of well being is not completely understood. Serotonin is also found in the gastrointestinal tract and plays a role in appetite and our perception of resources. For example, in response to the perception of abundance - meaning food - it can elevate mood; in response to scarcity, it can depress mood. It is thus associated with depression on a gut level, literally.

Serotonin is also associated with muscle contraction, and going deeper into the food-abundance-happiness connection, it may work in a seesaw relationship with dopamine. When humans smell food, dopamine is released to increase the appetite; serotonin is subsequently released to activate muscles used for feeding, which in turn halts the release of dopamine. Interestingly, serotonin is also associated with social rank. It has been observed that animals become dominant in a social setting when injected with serotonin, which may allow them to take food from weaker individuals. Serotonin has other properties as well. It is associated with cognitive functions, including memory and learning, and sleep as well as growth factors for some cells and cellular healing.

The main thing for us to know about serotonin is that higher levels lead to a feeling of happiness and help keep our moods under control by helping with sleep, calming anxiety, and relieving depression. Low levels lead to mild or moderate depression, anxiety, apathy, fear, feelings of worthlessness, insomnia, and fatigue. Most antidepressant drugs prevent the breakdown of serotonin.

DIETARY SOLUTIONS

The average person would be amazed at the number of drugs that are used to treat neurotransmitter deficiencies, or any of the depressions and anxieties that result. The problem with these drugs is that they don't really replenish the neurotransmitter; they only treat symptoms of the deficiencies.

This leads to the question of why we don't just inject neurotransmitters. The reason is because it doesn't work. The chemicals cannot cross what is known as the blood-brain barrier, a filter of sorts between the brain and its blood, designed to protect the neural environment. You've got to take something that crosses the blood-brain barrier and helps the brain manufacture the transmitter. Serotonin, for example, has to be manufactured in the brain. Otherwise we'd all be getting massive serotonin injections and walking around like happy idiots.

Instead we take antidepressant medications that are really serotonin re-uptake inhibitors (SRI), which leave more serotonin in the synapses. This is an artificial, synthetic way to attack the problem. Yes, people are walking around happier, but they are also zombies, with other side effects experienced. The question is, would you rather be just plain happy, or a happy zombie with side effects? Obviously we'd all rather just be happy, or brighter, or calmer, or able to achieve whatever benefit might come from a higher level of a given neurotransmitter. What is the best way to do that? Help your brain replenish its neurotransmitters naturally, and in a healthier way, through diet, supplements, and hormones.

REPLENISHING NEUROTRANSMITTERS

Neurotransmitters are manufactured in your body, but there are foods, supplements, and hormones that can help you achieve an environment conducive to their production and balance.

FOR ACETYLCHOLINE

FOODS:

- Almonds
- Artichokes
- Lean
- Beef
- Broccoli
- Brussels
- Sprouts
- Cabbage
- Egg
- Fish (especially cod, salmon, tilapia)
- Hazelnuts
- Liver (beef, turkey, chicken)
- Macadamia nuts
- Oat bran
- Peanut butter
- Pine nuts
- Pork
- Shrimp
- Soy protein powder

SUPPLEMENTS:

- Acetyl-L-carnitine
- Choline
- Deanol (DMAE)
- Fish oils
- Gingko biloba
- Huperzine-A
- Korean ginseng
- Linoleic acid
- Lipoic acid
- Manganese
- Pantothenic acid (Vitamin B5)
- Phosphatidylcholine
- Phosphatidylserine
- Taurine
- Thiamine
- Vitamin B12

HORMONES:

- Calcitonin
- DHEA
- Erythropoietin
- Estrogen
- Human growth hormone (HGH)
- Parathyroid hormone
- Vasopressin

FOR DOPAMINE

FOODS:

- Chicken
- Chocolate (dark)
- Cottage
- Cheese
- Duck
- Egg
- Granola
- Milk (whole only)
- Oat flakes or rolled oats
- Pork
- Ricotta
- Turkey
- Wheat germ
- Wild game
- Yogurt

SUPPLEMENTS:

- Vitamin B complex
- Ginkgo biloba
- Methionine
- Phenylalanine
- Phosphatidylserine
- Pyridoxine
- Rhodiola

HORMONES:

- Calcitonin
- Cortisol
- DHEA
- Erythropoietin
- Estrogen
- Human growth hormone (HGH)
- Prostaglandin
- Testosterone
- Thyroxine
- Vasopressin

FOR GABA

FOODS:

- Almonds
- Banana
- Beef liver
- Brown rice
- Citrus
- Halibut
- Lentils
- Oats, whole grain
- Potato
- Spinach
- Walnuts
- Whole wheat (and other whole grains)

SUPPLEMENTS:

- Glutamic acid
- Inositol
- Niacianamide (vitamin B3)
- Passionflower
- Pyridoxine (vitamin B6)
- Thiamine
- Valerian root

HORMONES:

- Melatonin

FOR SEROTONIN

FOODS:

- Avocado
- Banana
- Cheese
- Chicken
- Chocolate
- Cottage cheese
- Duck
- Egg
- Granola
- Luncheon meat
- Milk (whole only)
- Oat flakes
- Papaya
- Pork
- Ricotta
- Sausage meat
- Turkey (remember those happy Thanksgivings?)
- Wheat germ
- Wild game
- Yogurt

SUPPLEMENTS:

- Calcium
- Fish oils
- 5-HTP
- Magnesium
- Melatonin
- Passionflower
- Pyridoxine
- SAM-e
- St. John's wort
- Tryptophan
- Zinc

HORMONES:

- Adenosine
- Human growth hormone (HGH)
- Leptin
- Pregnenolone
- Progesterone

PHARMACEUTICAL SOLUTIONS (DRUGS)

As I mentioned, there are also a host of pharmaceutical solutions to the symptoms of low and imbalanced neurotransmitter levels. Many people go to psychiatrists or family practitioners for treatment of these symptoms. They are typically offered pharmaceutical solutions, and for these treatments to have a positive result, the prescribing physician must closely monitor the patient.

Very often, these doctors do not take the time to determine the root of the problem. Instead they just throw the drug at their patient as a solution without engaging or educating the patient, and sometimes without adequate follow-up to monitor, manage and adjust therapies as needed. A great deal of this is a result of the U.S. insurance companies. Sadly, they don't cover the type of visits that allow doctors to get to know their patients well enough to adequately treat them. This 'drive-thru' style of health care leaves physicians in a difficult position: they must either ignore the symptoms and hope for a time when they can more thoroughly examine the patient, refer them to a sub-specialist, or offer palliative care for the symptoms via a prescription. More often than not, the third choice is taken.

I am not in any way trying to disparage my medical colleagues. Unfortunately, though, the pharmaceutical ads, which are everywhere these days, are quite adept at making people think they can self-diagnose. They ask questions such as, "Ever feel sad?" Well, who doesn't feel sad from time to time? These medications don't diagnose or cure anything; they only mask the symptoms. This is why I practice anti-aging medicine, because my desire to help is focused on why something is happening and how we can deal with that cause.

This is not to say that pharmaceuticals do not have a place in health care. Some pharmaceuticals do help, at least for the short term, and there are patients who need that bridge. You can't turn your life around if you can't get out of your pajamas in the morning, and just as they couldn't turn the Titanic on a dime, patients' problems don't turn around overnight. Healing and progress take time, especially if trying to fix someone functionally using a more natural approach, like the lifestyle, dietary, and hormone balances we have been discussing. The goal, however, is to get off of chemical medication in a short period of time - a very realistic goal.

Many of the patients I see are already on antidepressants. This is no surprise. The number of Americans on antidepressants is astonishing, and it is the most commonly prescribed medication. Although the statistics are somewhat unclear, there are probably sixty million people on antidepressants at any given time, about one in five Americans. Baby Boomers, it seems, have inordinately high levels of depression.

One of the things I find myself doing, time after time, is weaning people off antidepressants. Once I help a patient get 'in balance', and we've addressed all the issues, there's no need for the prescription medication anymore. They're in balance, they're feeling good, and once off the meds they will no longer have side effects to worry about.

The problem with antidepressants is that they offer a quick fix in an era where depression is epidemic. We're living in a society in which Baby Boomers are aging and falling into that irritable syndrome, and with it, depression. Instead of dealing with it in a functional way, many people try to get by with a quick fix. They still have to work and live, and they don't know what else to do.

Part of the current antidepressant craze has to do with our culture. Aging in today's society is different than it was even one generation ago. There are more demands on older people than ever before, and thanks to our lost sense of community, people are feeling more alienated, afraid, and challenged at exactly the stage of life when they have earned the right to feel even more safe, secure, calm and comfortable than in earlier years when we are building our futures. This has led to the higher incidence of depression that I see too often.

We need to address these issues head-on, not with a pill that masks symptoms, but by looking deeper for a solution that ends the need for medication. Anything less comes from a lack of information, and a lack of apparent options. Today's medicine has been pushed on the public by pharmaceutical companies. This is unfortunate, because so much of what people suffer from can be treated through lifestyle change rather than by pills. Thankfully, this is beginning to change.

THE BRAIN/BODY CONTINUUM

It's important to understand the notion of the brain/body continuum, in which every physical state is reflected in a psychological state, and vice versa. Does this apply to brain chemicals? Is there a neurotransmitter relationship to basic bodily functions? If dopamine is related to energy, for example, and you become more physically energetic, do you create a higher dopamine level?

The answer is yes, yes, and yes. There is an important feedback loop here. What happens in your mood, your level of energy, and your sense of mental sharpness is reflected in the chemistry of your brain and the chemistry and functionality of your body, and it works in both directions. The positive effects of good diet, regular exercise, sufficient sleep, and a less stressful lifestyle all translate into changes in your neurotransmitter levels and therefore your mood.

As described earlier, patients with low dopamine levels generally develop terrible diets and poor lifestyles. They are typically plagued by hormone issues. These are interesting associations and you can see how they are related. If you have low dopamine levels, you're going to gain weight, which encourages poor lifestyle and leads to other biochemical issues, such as high cortisol levels and low sex hormones. It feeds back on itself and the cycle repeats. The behavioral issues, in turn, contribute to low dopamine levels.

It's all connected, especially when it comes to the effects of hormones. Memory loss or a mental fog can be caused by low dopamine and low acetylcholine, but low hormone levels also contribute, or are at least firmly associated. We have to look at all the various factors that influence cognition and mental processing time, and then look at how fast your brain is and examine what influences that speed. There are lots of different factors. Stress can put someone in a brain fog, as can depression or sleep deprivation. It boils down to how our biochemistry is influenced by what we ingest and how we act.

Other issues can alter your body and brain chemistry as well - taking it from homeostasis to unbalanced. These can include changes in your cortisol, insulin, and blood sugar levels, as well as your adrenalin and noradrenalin levels. All of these create different biochemical processes that are eventually going to affect neurotransmitters in your brain.

Hormone balance is an essential part of this equation. It is necessary for normal, balanced, biochemical functions, and to maintain normal neurotransmitter balance and cognitive clarity. There is no question that hormone levels have a significant influence, as will toxicities, food sensitivities, and allergies. All of these can be influencers, and lead to alteration of neural balance and brain chemistry.

Low levels of neurotransmitters and the depression and mental fog they create should be counteracted with diet, supplements, and hormone replacement - not pharmaceuticals.

Remember, while the brain clearly plays a preeminent role in how we feel and act, how we feel and act also translates into brain chemistry.

HAPPINESS AND LIVING WELL

There's a saying: "Living well is the best revenge." When it comes to anti-aging, this is not too far off the mark. The goal is to live a happy life. Any program that does not include a hefty serving of happiness has no chance of success.

As we discussed in the last chapter, negativity, in and of itself, is a barrier to success. It creates obstructions to improvements in wellness, vitality, and a longer health span. If you are negative, you are less likely to feel good. On the other hand, if you feel good, you are less likely to be negative.

http://www.youtube.com/watch?v=JPF mthpfNjc

One of the biggest challenges my patients face in their struggle to renew and rejuvenate themselves, is an obsession with perfection. These are people who have decided to change themselves, to start over, and there is a tendency to throw in the towel when they stumble. One of the best things I can impart is the idea that if you fall off the 'horse', get back on. For example, if you didn't follow your diet exactly one day, that doesn't mean you have to throw the whole thing out. Maybe you just had a bad day. It happens. Perhaps stress at work is getting to you and you revert back to some old habits, or you've reached a plateau and are taking a pause before moving on. Just because you have a chocolate bar or ice cream soda doesn't suddenly make you an obese person.

At the beginning of the program, I tell my patients not to be discouraged if they only accomplish a small amount at first. Any change in the right direction is vastly better than no change at all. The first few changes are going to have the biggest impact, especially for people who have been living an unhealthy lifestyle for a long time. For them, a little change goes a long way.

STRIKING THE RIGHT BALANCE

Have you noticed how the word 'balance' keeps reappearing in this book, chapter after chapter? Well, balance is what life is all about. The goal is to strike a balance between your physical, mental, and emotional health.

Once my patients are fully engaged in the anti-aging program. I try to instill the 'eighty/twenty formula'. I tell them that as long as they are doing the right thing eighty percent of the time, they'll be fine. It's all right to let it slide the other twenty percent of the time, because that may be what is needed to have fun in life. The idea is that you have to be happy on a regular basis. Any program that leaves you feeling miserable or worried most of the time, is going to fail.

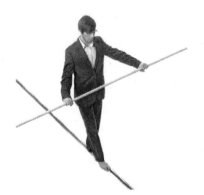

You're a human being, not a robot, and you shouldn't have to act like you are programmed a certain way. As a human, you have emotions, and you are going to slip up. You can't be one hundred percent, one hundred percent of the time, but as long as you can maintain the eighty/twenty balance, you are going to be successful.

Yes, there are those who can achieve one hundred percent, or at least very close to it. That's wonderful, - but such people are few and far between. We may all want to be this perfect person, but most of us hide certain things we do because we don't want to admit we're imperfect. We all have pleasures - secret and not-so-secret; the little indulgences that make life fun. If you can't enjoy these pleasures, life is a gray existence. The bottom line is that you can still enjoy life and reap all of the benefits of an anti-aging program as well.

Don't Be So Hard On Yourself

You don't have to be perfect to live well. You can actually live 'perfectly', and yet be miserable living that way. If you get on an anti-aging program and hate everything about it - the food, the discipline - it's not going to work. Most people have lived their lives in a very different way. They may hate the results of their lifestyle, but they liked the experience. In other words, they didn't get to the right destination - when they got there they were horrified - but they loved the ride. Now I'm telling you to take a different path, but if you can't stand the ride, it's not going to work.

People shouldn't be taught, instructed, or even encouraged to the point of being rigid. Just do eighty percent of it right, then take a day off and have that vanilla milk shake. Believe me, that eighty percent is going to change your life and you're going to be much, much better for it. No one is expecting you to be perfect. You're a human being, you have a brain, you have feelings, and you can have a bad day. Don't be so hard on yourself, because you can also get back on track the next day. You don't want to string those bad days along, of course, but once in a while you will make choices that aren't 'perfect' and that's okay, because being human means you are both fallible and resilient.

My philosophy at RVI is that we want people to be successful, and anything they can do towards that is good. Even if the effort is small and incremental, it's going to yield some improvement, and some improvement is far better than no improvement at all.

LOVE, AT LAST

Finally, when it comes to happiness and the achievement of a happy and joyous life, you cannot leave
out the importance of love and what it does for us.

http://www.youtube.
com/watch?v=jYK
eUmwTniM

Love may be the most studied and yet least understood
subject in the world. We truly don't understand what
it means, this whole idea of nurturing and affection.
There are so many aspects to the idea of love that it's almost impossible
to define. It is the single lyric that permeates almost all of popular
music, the single concept that drives most of our novels and movies,
and the reason most of us get up in the morning. Yet, we don't know
how it really works or even where it comes from.

I'll give you one small example. Just sit quietly, as comfortably as you
can, and breathe. Breathe deeply, not from up in your chest but from
the lower part of your stomach. Breathe in deeply and then take your
time breathing out. Do that for a minute, then close your eyes. Imagine
as hard as you can that all those breaths are going through your heart:
let them flow in and out through where you think your heart is.

After a while, you should feel a sensation. You'll get a feeling that
there is something real about the whole idea of the heart's connection
to the universe, and to the love that resides within you. This simple
exercise is just one tiny example of how much we don't understand
about love and the energy of the heart. It's a whole world of exploration
and comprehension unto itself.

I point this out because, in the hierarchy of life, love is definitely at
the top. Love is our center: it binds our relationships, spirituality, and
social connectivity. People who are part of strong social networks live
longer. These things give us purpose and help us deal with stress,
making them in turn fundamental to anti-aging.

This doesn't mean that I can tell you what love is, any more than I can tell you what spirituality means. It's a very complex thing, but we know that love is key to mitigating stress. Are there other aspects to love? Yes, there are many. Do we understand them? No. We're thinking more about it, and we're exploring it more, but right now I think the most useful thing to understand about love is that it makes you feel better, gives you a sense of direction, and helps reduce stress. The best way of putting it is that love is the best anti-aging therapy.

Love is the gateway to happiness. That is the point of this chapter and the entire book.

At its essence, anti-aging is the process of shedding bad habits that lead to bad living. It is the process of cleaning up our 'soup', and cleansing ourselves of the toxins in our food, water, and air. It is about coming closer to our natural selves; human beings who need the basics of exercise, nourishment, sleep, and social connectivity.

It is also about restoring the physiology of our metabolism and rejuvenating our systems with the chemistry of youth. In the end, it is about returning to a place that is more authentic and connected, both inside and outside, and through these exercises and interventions, to recreate a joyous youthfulness that allows us to lead purposeful, vital, and happy lives to the fullest extent possible well into our later years.

Good luck on your journey to a more youthful, happy self.

CHALLENGES TO YOUR PROGRAM

APPENDIX

Starting and maintaining the RVI anti-aging program is heroic enough, but there are challenges you may face that can present obstacles to your success. Being able to effectively hurdle these obstacles is what will ultimately make you the success you've worked so hard to be.

CHALLENGE 1: SMOKING

I am often asked if I would treat a smoker. I have to give a mixed answer. Part one is that if a patient will not quit smoking, the anti-aging program is never going to get them where they want to go. I won't decline working with them, at least not initially, but I'm going to keep pushing them to quit smoking. I want them to know that as long as they keep smoking it's going to undermine most of what we're doing to help them prevent the development of chronic disease. I can't protect them if they are smokers.

Fortunately, I see fewer and fewer smokers all the time. I see a lot of people who tell me they've already quit, and that is one of the best things they could ever do for their health. I tell patients who haven't quit that if they can quit, they'll be very successful with the program.

I admire people who have quit smoking, because that means they have overcome a really serious addiction. It's very empowering to do this, and I believe that people who quit smoking can do almost anything. Those who have quit are good candidates for the program. If they haven't quit yet, I try to help them finally do it.

First I try to figure out how willing they are, because you can't get somebody to quit who doesn't want to. I must determine whether or not they are committed, because if they are not committed to quitting, it's a waste of time trying. That's a prescription for a one hundred percent failure rate, so what's the point?

MOKING

Currently Smoking?	Yes No	How many years?		Packs per day:
Attempts to quit:				
Previous Smoking: How many years?			Packs per day:	
2nd Hand smoke exposure?				

ALCOHOL INTAKE

How many drinks currently per week?
1 drink = 5 ounces wine, 12 oz beer, 1.5 ounces spirits
☐ None ☐ 1-3 ☐ 4-6 ☐ 7-10 ☐ >10 If "None," skip to Other Substances

Previous alcohol intake?	Yes (Mild - Moderate - High) None
Have you ever been told you should cut down your alcohol intake?	Yes No
Do you get annoyed when people ask you about your drinking? Yes No	
Do you ever feel guilty about your alcohol consumption? Yes No	
Do you ever take an eye-opener? Yes No	
Do you notice a tolerance to alcohol (can you "hold" more than others)? Yes No	
Have you ever been unable to remember what you did during a drinking episode? Yes No	
Do you get into arguments or physical fights when you have been drinking? Yes No	
Have you ever been arrested or hospitalized because of drinking? Yes No	
Have you ever thought about getting help to control or stop your drinking? Yes No	

OTHER SUBSTANCES

Caffeine intake: Yes No	Cups/day:	Coffee Tea	☐ 1 ☐ 2-4 ☐ > 4 a day
Caffeinated Sodas or Diet Sodas Intake: Yes No			
12-ounce can/bottle/day: ☐ 1 ☐ 2-4 ☐ > 4 a day			
List favorite type: Ex. Diet Coke, Pepsi, etc.			
Are you currently using any recreational drugs? Yes No Type:			
Have you ever used IV or inhaled recreational drugs? Yes No			

Plan for Success

If they are committed to quitting smoking, I use different methods. In terms of a specific way to stop, I believe two things. First, I believe that anything that works is the way to go. Second, whether you slowly wind down or go cold turkey, I never tell a patient that they are going to quit tomorrow, as in the very next day. Instead I let them pick a date. It could be next week, next month, or in two months. I tell them to psych themselves up, and if they're committed, choose a date and stick with that date. That's when they are going to quit.

Then it becomes a planned event. It's all part of the idea that you have to plan things if you want them to happen. You have to have a goal in order to achieve a result. People are less likely to be successful when they don't plan, when they are impulsive. That leaves them exposed to influences that will distract and disrupt them from achieving their goal. It's the same thing with nutrition, exercise, stress reduction, or any other lifestyle change. If you plan ahead you can be successful because you will be more able to include good behaviors that will support reaching your goal, and avoid bad habits that will present obstacles or triggering factors you need to avoid. Planning fosters success.

I tell patients, "Pick a date, but once you pick it, that's your date. You own it. Now let's start planning for that date. What do you have to do to get yourself ready?" Some will try to reduce their smoking prior to that date, though I think a cold turkey approach is best.

Start Stopping

When the scheduled quitting date arrives, I like to start patients with something that helps them, but is easy. One way to go is the nicotine patch and nicotine gum, which reduce cravings. Another medication is a prescription pill called Chantix®, which is taken for the week before the date they are going to quit. I increase the dosage immediately following the day they stop, which also seems to reduce cravings. Wellbutrin® is another prescription drug that may sometimes be effective.

Another option that's been successful for many of my patients is the laser, where light-based lasers are used to stimulate certain meridians, usually around the ear lobes, which are associated with acupuncture points. This seems to work. I've sent many of my patients to a clinic that specializes in this technique, and surprisingly, we've seen a seventy-five to eighty-five percent success rate, which is pretty high.

The first thing I like to try, however, is cognitive behavioral therapy, since quitting is really about learning a new habit and healthy alternative coping behaviors. Cognitive behavioral therapy is focused on examining the cues that trigger the unhealthy behavior(s) and then teaching patients alternative healthy behaviors as coping mechanisms.

Another approach I like is hypnotism, which I have actually had a lot of success with. I send RVI patients to a hypnotherapist who knows how to do it well, someone who is experienced, skilled, and has a good track record. Of course, not everybody is a good fit for this treatment, and a good hypnotist will let you know if you are not a good subject. My feeling is that hypnotherapy doesn't hurt, and if it does work then it is very well worth it. In fact, if hypnotism works to break the smoking habit, I recommend that my patients use it for other habits as well, to help them achieve and maintain a healthier lifestyle.

The important thing is quitting, so you do what's necessary. Many people may fail on their first attempt, but they must continue to try, and if they keep trying, eventually there is a reasonable chance they will succeed.

I've had many patients who tried to quit smoking and failed. My conclusion is that they were not truly ready to quit. They thought and said they were ready, but in the end it was revealed that they weren't, and that's probably why they failed. My approach is then to say, "Don't be discouraged; let me know when you're ready to try again. When you're committed to trying again, we'll do it again." Lo and behold, on their second, third or fourth try, they achieve success; but it has to be their number one priority. It comes down to understanding that nothing is more important - not any meeting, not any event. Nothing. It's that important to quit. Plain and simple, smoking ages you and then it kills you.

CHALLENGE 2:
SUGAR, INSULIN SENSITIVITY & DIABETES

When it comes to nutrition and diet, Americans today are mostly concerned with fatty foods. We are worried about fat in our food because we've been taught to worry about cholesterol, and because we are worried about being or becoming fat ourselves.

What we should be worried about is sugar. Sugar is the new fat! It is more dangerous than fat, and more destructive. It is, in fact, deadly. Sugar is a killer and I will tell you why.

If I were on a desert island and I had only one test I could take to see how healthy I was, or how long I had to live, it would be the test for what's called the 'fasting level' of insulin. This is the most important level you can measure, because it measures your level of insulin resistance.

To understand how deadly sugar is, we have to take a quick look at how sugar and insulin interact, and what causes diabetes. This is how it works:

Insulin Sensitivity (and Sugar)

Insulin is a hormone produced by the pancreas. It is produced to deal with the sugar in your bloodstream and do something with it. Every time we eat and digest food, we release glucose (i.e. sugar) into our bloodstream. Our pancreas senses that sugar and produces insulin, which in turn tells our cells that it's time to eat. Receptors on the cells 'catch' the insulin, which then stimulates the cells to absorb the sugar. If there is more glucose in the bloodstream than your cells actually need, your body stores away the excess for future energy needs. The glucose is stored in one of two ways, either as fat or as something called glycogen, which is stored in the liver. This glucose will later be released in a measured way to fill our energy needs, when there is no more glucose in the blood, but for now it is packed away in your fat cells and liver.

This continues until there is a low (i.e. normal) amount of glucose in the blood, at which time the pancreas stops producing insulin. So think of insulin as the traffic cop that decides how each fresh energy supply of glucose is processed by the human body.

Hold on, that is only part of the story. Insulin, and your sensitivity to it, also determines how efficiently you use that energy. If your cells have a normal sensitivity to glucose, all is well, but if your cells have been exposed to too much insulin too many times - thanks to all the sugar that you dump into your system, way more than your body was evolved to handle - then your cells start to develop what is called insulin resistance. They don't respond properly to all that insulin, and don't absorb all that sugar.

The consequence of this insulin resistance is that you will have too much unabsorbed glucose in your blood. Your body tries to do something with it, which typically means turning it into extra fat. That's why our sugar-rich nation is so overweight and why a measurement of our resistance to insulin is so important. It gets even worse, however. With our sugar-rich diets, there can be so much glucose in our blood over an extended period of time that the body can't clear it out. It builds up in your system, and you end up with chronically high levels of glucose that can cause significant health problems.

One result is damage to your tissues, because the chronic presence of all that glucose causes accelerated cellular rust, which is another term for inflammation. Chronic inflammation is associated with a host of diseases, from rheumatoid arthritis to lupus to atherosclerosis to Alzheimer's, just to name a few, and inflammation is very closely connected to insulin resistance.

In the short term, however, excess chronic glucose in the blood mainly causes obesity - and diabetes.

Diabetes, Defined

There are two types of diabetes. **Type 1** and **Type 2.**

Type 1 diabetes is typically developed in childhood and results from an autoimmune response in your body. Your immune system treats the insulin-producing beta cells in your pancreas as foreign objects, and destroys them. Without insulin to tell your cells that it's time to eat, your cells starve.

Type 2 diabetes is also called adult-onset diabetes because it develops in adulthood. Basically, it occurs when your cells develop such insensitivity to insulin that no matter how much is over-produced by the pancreas, your cells simply don't respond. Their insulin receptors have gone numb. The result, again, is cellular starvation in the midst of plenty.

Type 2 diabetes is a challenge we are often faced with in anti-aging. It's usually the result of weight gain, which is caused by chronic ingestion of processed foods and sugar and too many calories. As noted above, this surplus over time has caused you to pump out more insulin to control and deal with excess sugar, which causes resistance to the insulin that is working well. Meanwhile you keep pumping out more insulin to deal with excess sugar, until one of two things happens; either your pancreas gets tired and can't keep it up, or you get so resistant to insulin that no matter how much you're pumping out, it still can't do the job.

When this happens, the result will be sustained high blood sugar levels combined with an inability to utilize that sugar effectively - or to effectively deal with the mobilization of the stored sugar in your fat, which is something else that insulin does. If this happens you are definitely going to have energy issues.

How To Test for Diabetes

I monitor this in two basic ways. The traditional method is to measure the 'fasting' blood sugar level. If your blood sugar level is chronically high, then you are somebody who potentially has an issue with clearing the sugar from your system.

Another test is called hemoglobin A1c. This test tells you how your glucose level has been over time. If it's been high over a prolonged period of time, then your hemoglobin A1c will be elevated. The more elevated it is, the more elevated your blood sugar has been over time. This is probably the most important test used today to diagnose diabetes.

Probably the most sensitive test is measurement of your fasting insulin level. Your fasting insulin level is important especially at the early stages of diabetes, before the pancreas is burned out. If you are pumping out a lot of insulin to deal with all the extra sugar stimulation in the presence of insulin resistance, then your fasting insulin rises. This is a clear sign that there is a problem.

The only weakness in this test is that, over time, when you exhaust your pancreas' insulin producing capabilities, you can have a situation where you measure your insulin level when you're fasting and it may actually be normal or low, but this may be a false indication of what is actually going on. In this case you have to stimulate your pancreas to produce insulin and then measure to see how it performs. This is called a glucose tolerance test with insulin, and it's what I do for most of my patients who have blood sugar problems. I have the patient consume a sugary drink. I take their fasting blood sugar and insulin level before they do this, and then measure fasting blood sugar and insulin levels every hour on the hour for 3 to 5 hours. If they are having a normal insulin response, it clears the sugar out in a normal fashion, but if they have an abnormal response, I can usually figure out their problem, and how to help.

Repairing the Damage

Again, the problems come down to either some level of insulin resistance, or an inability to produce insulin, which means the pancreas is impaired. The good news is that the situation doesn't have to be permanent, and most people can definitely come back from it, unless they've totally destroyed their ability to produce insulin - but that takes a long time of not doing anything about it. Most patients can get off of insulin-regulating medications by changing their lifestyle. It's all about diet, exercise, and balance.

In the meantime we do help the patients with certain medications that reduce insulin resistance, making it less of a factor. That's helpful, because it's very difficult for people to lose weight if they have insulin resistance.

In some cases insulin itself is needed, because when people have very high blood sugar, diet and exercise take time to be effective. I don't want these patients to reach a point where the blood sugar is so high that it's an imminent danger to their life. In these circumstances, if left untreated, it could lead to a life-threatening situation. In such cases I put them on insulin to get them down to a reasonable level, and then implement these other remedies to wean them off of insulin over time as they lose weight.

The most important treatment when the patient is overweight is to get them to a normal weight, and the most important treatment for people who are not overweight is to keep them on a calorie-controlled diet while encouraging them to exercise regularly.

This is why I would want a fasting insulin level test on a desert island. If someone has a high fasting insulin level, it means the blood sugar is chronically high and the body is chronically pumping out high levels of insulin, even while not eating.

By the way, since too much sugar begets too much insulin, which wears out receptors and burns out the pancreas, longevity depends on a lifelong low glucose level. That's why we know, with a very high degree of certainty, that caloric restriction is the one thing that will definitely increase longevity. The reason is that caloric restriction is associated with lower glucose levels, and hence high insulin sensitivity.

The bottom line here is to eat less, avoid sugars, and stick to whole foods, i.e. nature's foods. Whole food carbohydrates have generally high levels of natural fiber. This is very important because it slows down the absorption of glucose into the bloodstream, keeping your level of glucose at a lower and more constant, normal, ideal level.

CHALLENGE 3: WATER AND ALCOHOL

The easiest way to illustrate the importance of water versus food is in the absence of them. Go without water and you'll die in a matter of days. Go without food and you can easily last more than a month.

We are creatures of water; it comprises more than ninety percent of our body mass. So, logically, the consumption of water is vital to our existence, as well as our health.

One old wives tale of complexion is that drinking a lot of water is good for your skin. It certainly makes sense; nothing purifies and detoxifies our bodies on a daily basis more than the consumption of water, and drinking a lot of it is something I always recommend to my patients.

Personally, I drink a lot of water. It has become a habit, just like avoiding the sun. The general rule of thumb is that you should drink a half-ounce daily for every pound of weight. So, if you weigh one hundred pounds, you should be drinking fifty ounces, or about a liter and a half of water daily. If you weigh one hundred and fifty pounds, that would make it seventy-five ounces, or two liters and another eight-ounce glass (there are 33.76 fluid ounces in a liter). For a person weighing over two hundred pounds, that means three liters a day.

That may seem like a heck of a lot of water, but it doesn't all have to come from a line of eight-ounce glasses lined up on your counter, staring you in the face each day. You automatically get water from other sources, like fruits and vegetables, as well as from more obvious liquid sources like soup, tea, or other beverages.

To compensate, one question I am often asked about anti-aging is the proper amount of alcohol consumption. While alcohol is obviously made with water, it should not figure into your daily water consumption. Generally speaking, alcohol is a wonderful thing for most people if used correctly and not to excess. What does that mean? It means that alcohol used in moderation has a lot of proven health benefits. Red wine, the star of the show, has been shown to contain an array of antioxidants, the best known being Resveratrol. A glass or two of red wine daily is a key component of the Mediterranean diet, and is one of the probable causes of the good cardiac health associated with those who practice it. Moreover, alcohol is a relaxant that makes you feel good. It allows for positive social connectivity, not only in terms of social gatherings but also in terms of religious and cultural traditions. The importance of this cannot be dismissed.

On the other hand, alcohol can be addicting. You have to take this in context, especially if you have an addictive personality. Obviously I do not encourage people to drink if they have the potential of becoming addicted to alcohol, which is not uncommon.

Alcohol also contains a lot of calories, so a trade off is required. If you want to drink even one or two glasses of alcohol daily, and are weight challenged, you are going to have to make some trades and give up some calories somewhere else, in order not to put on the pounds. Otherwise, if you drink a couple of glasses of wine per night, that could add two hundred and fifty or so calories to your daily total, which is substantial.

Finally, alcohol has a negative effect on sleep for a lot of people, especially if consumed right before bed. This may seem counter-intuitive and a little unfair, since as a relaxant it can get you to the point of sleep, but once you fall asleep it can negatively influence sleep patterns, especially if you have a tendency toward obstructive sleep apnea.

Nonetheless, with these caveats in mind, I think alcohol can be beneficial, so long as it is consumed moderately and responsibly. From a health perspective we believe today that a little alcohol on a regular basis is beneficial, and while there is some benefit from any form of alcohol, such as beer or scotch, clearly red wine is the way to go. In terms of research, the most valid studies on the benefits of alcohol all point to wine as the best. In terms of quantity guidelines, for men the recommendation is up to two glasses of wine per day, and for women up to one.

Everyone should drink less if consuming spirits.

ANTI-AGING TRAVEL & PLANNING

Traveling is a big problem for any anti-aging prescription, especially air travel. Travel is flat out disruptive to normal physiology, yet today we live in a society where travel is common. I see the effects in my patients all the time, people who are part of the entertainment industry or have businesses around the country. They travel frequently - as do many other people who don't think twice about hopping on an airplane for work. I don't have to tell you how stressful air travel is. You're going through security, getting on airplanes, passing through time zones, rushed constantly, and then (unless seated in first class with people pampering you), you're crammed in like a sardine.

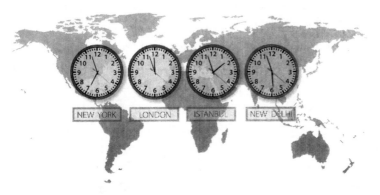

Once most people reach their destination they start working, and don't take time to go to the gym, or don't stay in a hotel that has a gym, or they're in business meetings at lunch and dinner, and everybody is drinking. Forget about maintaining a good diet while traveling; once most people are at restaurants, they lose control. The only thing harder on your diet than traveling, is traveling frequently.

Maintaining your anti-aging protocol requires planning to be successful even under these circumstances. I try to help my patients find other solutions. Planning is the key to travel. Think through your trip ahead of time and plan strategies to satisfy the basics of food, exercise, sleep and stress mitigation.

With travel what's important to understand, is that while you are leaving home, you are not leaving yourself. You take yourself with you wherever you go, which means taking your new habits and your new approach to living along as well, to be applied wherever you land.

If you don't have a plan, you will always be in a situation where you're going to default to whatever is available, based on whatever is happening to you in the moment. That's when you're vulnerable. For example, if one of your issues is diet, bring along good food instead of eating fast food, or research healthy restaurants before you go, so you can avoid that vulnerability. Think this through for every trip, and you won't be left without options.

Plan your other anti-aging habits for when you travel, as well. Create an exercise plan that takes into account your schedule; find running routes and/or schedule gym time. If you need to de-stress, then you need a de-stress plan, maybe something to satisfy your cultural or spiritual needs. Plan carefully and approach this 'homework' as part of your adventure, ways to stay healthy and youthful in a new location. When you invest the time in staying committed to this journey, you won't be left without options while away, and you'll be less likely to let yourself down. Schedule some quiet time, go to a play, or visit a museum. Otherwise, you either won't do anything at all, or you'll fall back on old, harmful behaviors.

Think of planning as anti-aging behavioral modification, reprogramming yourself to form and maintain new habits. Indeed, we find it common among our patients that forming new anti-aging habits is virtually impossible without planning, and without integrating a plan into each day. This is particularly apparent when we travel because our routines are already disrupted.

In terms of how to travel under the anti-aging banner, I give my patients specific ideas. In general, I suggest doing everything possible to minimize the stress of the experience, because it's going to be stressful no matter what. Still, you can mitigate much of this stress. For example, allow yourself enough time to minimize the stress of travel. It sounds like common sense, and it is, but that doesn't mean people practice it automatically. If you think of the factors that stress people out about travel, a major one is the rush of it. So, don't rush! Don't leave things to the last minute. Take your time, get there early, and reduce stress.

Another thing you can do is plan your nutrition ahead of time. If you're getting on a flight where they don't serve food, bring your own. Buy water for the airplane, as dehydration is common on long flights. Closely related to this is your restaurant diet. I often tell patients what they're supposed to eat, so when they go to a restaurant they'll know what to do. Nothing changes because you're at a restaurant. If everybody's drinking over dinner, then have a glass of red wine. Don't deprive yourself; just stick to the plan as much as possible.

Next, if you are crossing time zones, you need to understand how that's going to throw you off. You don't want to disrupt your circadian rhythms, so you should prepare by making little adjustments ahead of time. If you are traveling west, it's going to be relatively later on your internal clock when you get there, so I advise patients to make the adjustment by going to bed later one or two nights before departure. If you are traveling east, your internal clock is going to be relatively earlier than when you get there, so you should adjust ahead of time by going to sleep earlier.

Melatonin is useful in this regard, to adjust your clock. You can take melatonin when you're ready to sleep in your new destination, and that will help adjust your clock. If you take it at that time a day before you leave, even better. If you arrive in the evening at your location (typically going east) you need to get some melatonin in your system and get to bed sooner rather than later. If you arrive in the morning at your location (typically going west) you don't want to go to sleep. Try to get in bright light immediately and stay there. These things will help you adjust faster to the time shift.

Speaking of bright, ambient, full-spectrum light, I suggest that my patients bring a portable full-spectrum lighting device with them. This is for those situations when they can't get out and take a stroll or experience natural full-spectrum lighting for an extended period of time. In such cases it really helps if they can take a small full-spectrum light with them and turn it on, letting it shine on their face for half an hour. It's a simple thing, but it makes a difference because we are programmed to be exposed to sunlight.

Finally, I tell my patients to get some exercise. If there is no gym, then go for walk, wherever you are. If there is a gym, use it. This is very important, because the big problem with travel is that while people are under the impression that they are in motion, they're actually more sedentary when they travel. They sit in an airplane for hours, then go to a hotel and lie down, or sit in business meetings, or sit in cabs. Get moving whenever and wherever possible. You'll be better off for it.

I go through an exercise inventory with RVI patients, to help them understand how much or little they are actually moving when they travel. Typically there isn't much exercise, but there are big meals and increased alcohol consumption. On top of this, many people don't sleep well when they travel, and all of this leads to negative effects. I remind patients to do the right thing, because that's what will mitigate the aging effects of modern travel.

ACKNOWLEDGMENTS

This book was always meant to be the start of a series. My vision for The Beverly Hills Anti-Aging Prescription was to share my program for living a longer, more vital life by making improvements in several areas that I outline in the book. I have always felt that we need to take advantage of the years we have because they are finite, and I wanted to share my insights with a larger audience than just my patients. I hope that after reading The Beverly Hills Anti-Aging Prescription, you feel the same inspiration that my patients feel when they come see me in my office to get started on the path toward a healthier way of life.

There were many people involved in putting this book together and making its publication a reality.

A special thanks to J.P. Faber - my co-author, my assistant Ileanna Portillo and Rachael Martin who coordinated and organized all the tasks that contributed to the bigger picture.

CPSIA information can be obtained at www.ICGtesting.com
Printed in the USA
LVOW12s1055131113

361057LV00011B/357/P

9 780741 497178